EMBODY YOUR MAGIC

Create the Life of Your Dreams Through Astrology, Numerology, Mediumship, Metaphysics, and Human Design

EMBODY YOUR MAGIC

AYCEE BROWN

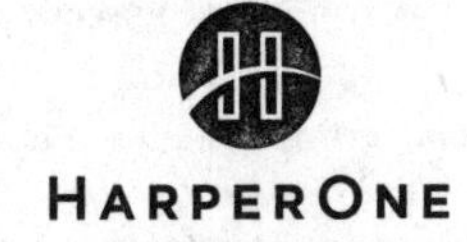

HarperOne
An Imprint of Harper Collins*Publishers*

The names and identifying characteristics of some of the individuals featured throughout this book have been changed to protect their privacy.

The material on linked sites referenced in this book is the author's own. HarperCollins disclaims all liability that may result from the use of the material contained at those sites. All such material is supplemental and not part of the book. The author reserves the right to close the website in their sole discretion at any time.

 For information, address HarperCollins Publishers, 195 Broadway, New York, NY 10007. In Europe, HarperCollins Publishers, Macken House, 39/40 Mayor Street Upper, Dublin 1, D01 C9W8, Ireland.

HarperCollins books may be purchased for educational, business, or sales promotional use. For information, please email the Special Markets Department at SPsales@harpercollins.com.

harpercollins.com

FIRST EDITION

Designed by Bonni Leon-Berman

Illustrations © Jill Allyn Peterson

Library of Congress Cataloging-in-Publication Data has been applied for.

ISBN 978-0-06-336032-7

Printed in the United States of America

25 26 27 28 29 LBC 5 4 3 2 1

To my younger self

and all the parts

that protected her

Contents

The Start of Your Journey:

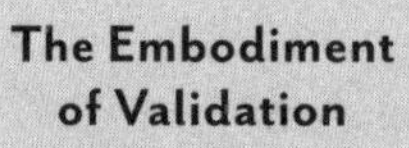

The Embodiment of Validation

Knowing Your Story

Who Am I?

Exiled Parts

The Embodiment of Anger

Psychic Channeling

When Did I Get Influenced?

Firefighter Parts

The Embodiment of Self

Astrology

Where Can I Surrender in My Life and Allow Ease?

The Self

The Embodiment of Alignment

Numerology

What's Not Aligning in My Life, Business, or Career?

Manager Parts

Embracing the Unknown

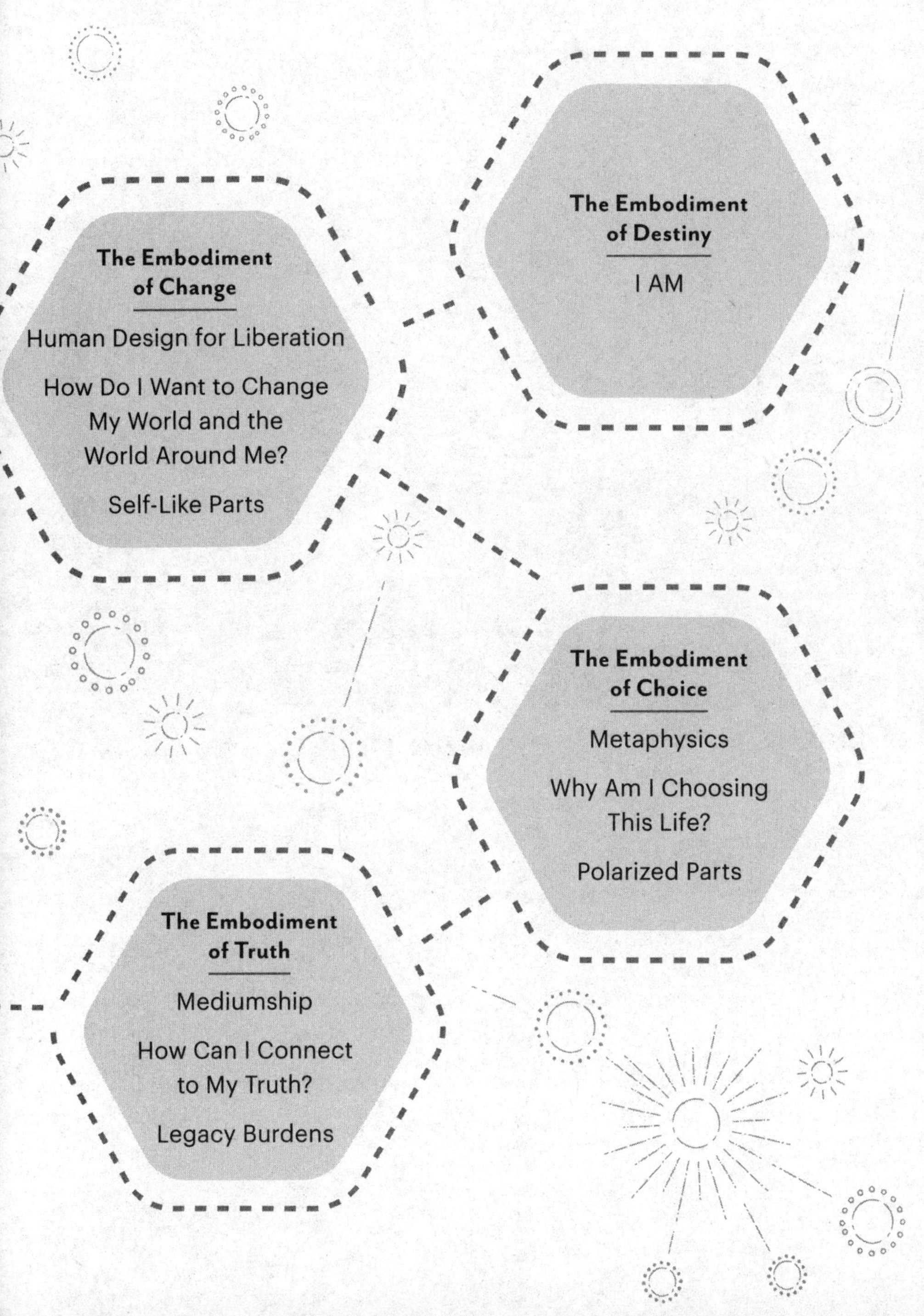

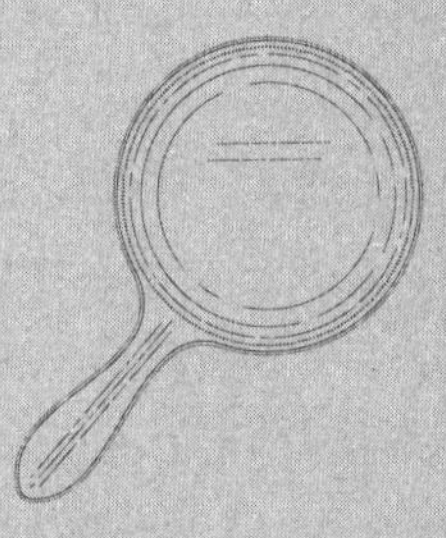

Are you ready to accept the journey? Circle Yes or No.

THE START OF YOUR JOURNEY

Embracing the Unknown

YOU'RE AT A CROSSROADS, and it's you and your old self looking each other in the eyes, both on the verge of tears, knowing that one of you must let go. The person who must let go is the new you. The healed version of you. The you after multiple therapy sessions. The you who wants more for yourself than you've been conditioned to believe you can have. The problem is you don't know how to say goodbye. The old version of yourself has protected you and kept you safe from harm. Your old version helped you create the walls that kept you safe from inner child wounds, untrustworthy family and friends, lovers who scorned you, and environments that seemed okay but turned out to be toxic.

You must look the old you in the eyes and thank them and say goodbye because they have gotten you as far as you could go together. Before you let go, you must forgive the person you used to be; it's the only way to walk a new path to the life you truly desire. It's time to draw a line in the sand and look back with a new perspective. Forgiving the person you used to be is one of the hardest things you'll ever do. It's not because you *want* to hold on to your old behaviors. It's because those behaviors saved your life at times when you needed to be saved. Your old self operated in unhealthy families, unhealthy careers, and unhealthy relationships. The person you used to be helped you become who you are today. They built your character and helped you learn lessons about yourself that no teacher could teach you.

They deserve your loyalty for helping you make it through those storms. It may have been your duty to soldier up and ride into the battlefields with your old self. But when the war is over or it's time to wave your white flag, the most loyal thing you can do is to thank yourself and grow. You no longer must fight for your life. You survived, and now it's time to thrive. Now it's time to step into your calling. Now it's time to go after your dream career. Now it's time to live a life that's made for TV. This all is possible after you forgive your old self so you're able to step into You 2.0 fully and unapologetically.

What does that look like? It's a life where we don't just wake up and get into our routine and start the day. Instead, it's one where we are fueled by our soul's desire. We are motivated by who we are on this earth, and in these bodies, to learn. We are living into and through the depths of our souls. I used to think when I was at the lowest points of my life that god/spirit hated me because how could they let this happen to me? But as I journeyed through life, I came to understand that things weren't happening to me—they were happening *for* me. I use the term *spirit* primarily to identify the energies and entities I have experienced beyond our three-dimensional lives, but please know, whatever form energy takes for you, and however you define it, is your true experience.

For my learning, for my healing, for my growth, these experiences acted as a balm for my soul's mending, so my spirit could flourish. Each moment, each challenge, was divinely orchestrated to expand my consciousness, mend the fragmented pieces of my being, and nurture my growth into the fullest expression of my potential. I would say that I didn't ask to be here when, actually, my spirit chose this. Now some might argue, *What about the really horrible shit?* No one would choose that. And I agree I didn't choose the trauma and abuse, but I did get to choose how I used those experiences to find and grow into the current version of myself. I chose to forgive my past self for doing what she needed to do to survive.

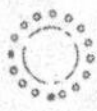

I RECENTLY VISITED BRISTOL CAVERNS IN Bristol, Tennessee. It was filled with crystals and had the acoustics of the best-sounding church, but it was also cold and dark. It was challenging to walk through. I had to climb up man-made stairs to see some parts, and the air quality was touch and go at times. The insides of the caves were fascinating. Touching the walls felt surreal; the minerals that had been produced over the centuries made them slippery yet beautiful.

By the end of it, I was ready to leave and breathe. It's hard to live in the canyons of our lives, and yet, we must go through it to emerge on the other side, to recognize that there are multiple points of entry and exit in our journey. There are ways into and around the canyons, but when we avoid them, we miss the beauty of life.

I want you to think about the canyon as your shadow. It's the deepest place you will ever be—the scariest, the most unknown—but it also holds your greatest reward. It holds the keys to your destiny. It holds the key to your vision, your voice, your "I AM."

Because on the other side of that pain is your most magical motherfucking life.

Discovering the Psychic Within

ONE DAY WHEN I WAS IN kindergarten, my mother and I were waiting at the bus stop when I pointed to a man and said as the bus pulled up, "Wait, that could be my father."

My mother paused and looked at me as if she had seen a ghost. "What are you talking about?" she said, shaking me off. "Your dad is your father."

At that time, I had no clue that the man I called Dad *wasn't* actually my father, but I knew that I knew things without other people having to tell me. When I was growing up in Queens, New York, my cousins and family called me scary. I would get a feeling about something, and many people would be so surprised that I would be right, even without knowing the details. Later, my grandmother began to see that I had a special gift, and she would have me help her with her "numbers," and with my help, she would always win the local lottery. As I grew older, she was the only one who I could confide in about my visions and dreams, which she quickly recognized made me special.

I could feel voices guiding me, but it took me years to realize that those voices were real—and that if I listened really closely, they were always right.

After years of pain and fear and, finally, deep work, I began to accept and even love these gifts. I spent a long time denying (and trying to ignore) the voices in my head. I thought I was going crazy. But through therapy and many more years learning to trust the voices, I found out that what I was hearing was real. But more important, I began to trust myself. The path to true psychic intuition requires us to trust ourselves more than we ever have before.

When I tell people they are psychic, they automatically think that means they're suddenly going to be seeing dead people, but that couldn't be further from the truth (although cheers to you if you do—spirits can offer some powerful guidance). No, true psychic ability is about connecting with all the teachings of the universe in order to be able to better understand this lifetime and our role within it. Though many people have dibbled and dabbled in psychic channeling, astrology, numerology, mediumship, human design, and metaphysics, often separately or at separate times throughout life, they have often walked away wondering why these avenues of healing or change didn't stick—or why they were still stuck. The easiest way to heal is to start our work knowing that healing is layered, that we will be triggered along the way because healing is hard, and that we won't get far without the tools to work our way through the darkest and deepest parts of ourselves. When we unravel the layers of our trauma personally, generationally, and ancestrally we unlock a direct connection to source/spirit/god. Once we tap into the hidden realms of our souls, we grant ourselves permission to embody our psychic abilities, allowing us to breathe life into this life and to turn our surviving into thriving.

As I began to hone my own skills, I realized that in order to truly embody the psychic within, I had to use all the tools available to me—my origin story, psychic channeling, astrology, numerology, mediumship, metaphysics, and human design—but it wasn't about trying a little bit of this or a little bit of that. It was about deep study, so I could braid them together into a tool kit that we can all access and use to embody the psychic within.

So, what is psychic ability? It's not just seeing the future or having a "sixth sense." Rather, it's feeling, knowing, and receiving things that cannot be explained by natural laws. When you get a feeling in the pit of your stomach that tells you something is not right, warns you not to go somewhere or engage with someone, or suggests that your partner is cheating, your soul is offering you truths that cannot be explained by natural laws. You are already psychic; however, your wounds block you from feeling, knowing, and receiving wisdom that cannot be explained by natural law. Embodying your magic is more about connecting to your truest self. Trusting the psychic within becomes a by-product of your healing. It gets you closer to your soul and your purpose here on earth.

The practices and tools that you will learn in this book aren't here just to split you open like a deli sandwich. They will also give you the tools to feast on the layers of magic and wonder that make up your life. The canyon is about embodying our destiny. The canyon symbolizes the deep and sometimes challenging journey each of us undertakes to fully embody our destiny. Just as a canyon is formed by the persistent flow of a river over a long period of time, carving out its unique path through the landscape, our lives are shaped by our experiences, our choices, and the inner currents of our desires and dreams.

Though it is often mistaken for mere darkness, the canyon is a realm of transcendent beauty—a sacred space where our true destiny unfolds. This isn't about recognizing the beauty that resides within our darkest moments; it's about fully embodying our divine path. It's the understanding that each shadow we encounter is not a hazard but a magical portal to our deepest transformation. The canyon is not for us to just walk through, admire what we see, or look at from afar. It calls us to touch the roughness, climb into the little crevices, and discover the glorious crystals inside: the gems that have been hidden for so long, maybe even as long as we can remember. But no matter where we begin the journey, whether at the beginning or further down in the canyon, we have an opportunity to claim our destiny, look at the parts that make us feel broken, and finally become our full selves.

The psychic channels are pathways to healing because they give us the opportunity to tackle many areas of our lives using different tools. Healing is not one-size-fits-all. It is very nuanced and can look different for each of us. But healing always starts with the truth, and the truth is hard. For many of us, it is easier to ignore what happened to us and what we went through to survive. How many times have you blocked out memories just to subdue your racing thoughts? But you can only do that for so long. When we start to uncover our traumas, we open issues that may never be resolved as quickly as we might want them to be.

Navigating into the depths of our truths isn't just a journey; it's the greatest gift we could ever give our future selves. This path, intertwined from the threads of our experiences, luminous and deeply shadowed, isn't about self-discovery; it's a pathway toward your soul's authenticity. I've come to realize that embracing your truth in its wholeness and fullness is the foundation to your soul's evolution. This journey is sacred because it brings light to the many hidden parts that we never knew existed. It's the ultimate act of self-love. And it's a tribute to your resilience, a bridge to your innermost self.

This journey through the canyon is a doorway to a future where you stand in your full power. I have always reminded myself that this exploration is not just about finding yourself but about creating yourself where you can thrive. When you dive into your truth, you get a chance to honor your past, embrace your present, and sculpt your future full of potential. In this exploration, we gift ourselves freedom of authenticity, strength in our convictions, and the beauty of our unpolished reality.

How to *Do* This Book

FIRST THINGS FIRST. THIS IS NOT a book you read. So, if you plan on just *reading* it, put this shit down right now. This is a book you *do*. It is a self-study guide to healing yourself. This book's purpose and promise are that when you finish it, you will finally know yourself. You will have references to look back to, and say, *Oh dear, this is why I make decisions the way I do*, or *This is how I feel when people hurt me*. You will have a self-study guide to assist you over and over as you grow and encounter new challenges. You also need to know that some parts of this book might take time.

Doing the work might reveal things that you've never known about yourself, or you might dig up more than you can manage. If that is the case, take this book with you when you go to your therapy or life coaching sessions. This isn't work you should do alone. Reach out to a trusted friend or family member who can hold you accountable. Think about embarking on this journey together and setting intentions to connect regularly about your progress. It's important to remember that you don't have to share every intricate detail of what you're discovering. The real value lies in offering emotional support and being a source of encouragement for each other. Focus on being present and uplifting one another, rather than getting caught up in all the nuances of each other's paths.

Be forewarned: It's not going to be easy, but within you lies an incredible power—the unshakable strength to journey through this path.

The psychic within, a deeply trusted and intuitive guide, is ready to cast a brilliant light on your way. Embrace this adventure wholeheartedly, for the wisdom nestled within your soul acts as both your compass and your guiding star, leading you with unwavering confidence toward the essence of your true self. Your spirit is your navigator, steering you toward your authentic truth with clear conviction.

Some people say the truth will set you free, but what they leave out is that the truth also fucking hurts. When we are born and start to journey through life, we each carry a set of questions that we need to answer in this lifetime. These questions guide our experiences, assist us in building relationships, and give us the tools to help heal our traumas. Sometimes the work is rainbows-and-sprinkles fun, but other times it can feel cold like ice or hot like a heat rash between your thighs. But it will clear up and go away over time. Just like your pain.

I believe one of our biggest misconceptions about this human experience is that we get dropped off on earth and are left to fend for ourselves. Often my clients will ask me, "Aycee, why would I have chosen this life? Why would my soul want to experience the pain, struggle, trauma, or challenging transitions that I constantly grow through?" I look them in the eyes and reply, "Because there was a lesson here that you still haven't learned from the last lifetime."

As you do this work, you will find yourself repeating patterns unlearned from your ancestral lineage, carrying forward the echoes

of your ancestors' experiences as if they were your own. This cycle of choices and consequences feels like a legacy of responsibilities and roles, a form of choose your own adventure handed down through the ages, where each generation takes its turn, perhaps in hopes of healing or breaking free from what came before. I think of this choice like shift work. I believe our lives are posted in the break room up above, and we look on the board and choose the type of experiences we want, what will fulfill our desires, and what we want to heal. And those shifts equate to certain lessons or healing experiences.

We are guided into our families, relationships, careers, friendships, and experiences to learn, grow, and heal in this lifetime. I began to realize that I wasn't alone in life, that none of us are. There is someone protecting us in the most subtle ways, whether we understand it or not.

Your soul has soldiers walking with you when you think you are alone.

Pause for a moment and recall an instance where you were caught in a challenging situation, wondering how you would ever navigate your way out of this temporary slump. In that moment of uncertainty, an intuitive nudge—a quiet yet compelling inner voice—prompted you to make a decisive move: to walk away from a place that no longer felt right, to end a relationship that was no longer serving you, or to start the search for a new professional beginning. This guidance, almost like a gentle push from the universe, was your soul's way of steering you toward the next chapter of your journey.

These little signs and nudges are the universe's way of letting you know that everything is working for your highest good, whether you see that or not. And as you will find, your ancestors are always there to carry the messages to you, if you are willing to receive them.

The questions that I was guided toward along this journey were hard to ask because I thought I knew the answers, but I was wrong. Once I started traveling down into my canyon, I had to be open to receive what spirit had to say to me. Through the years of honing my gifts and healing at the same time, many questions came up, but the one that came up at first was, *Who am I?* That question really came about because of the lingering question of my birth father. There were so many unknowns about him. That's when I started to hear from spirit louder, and I got a clear picture of who I was when I connected to spirit. I once thought there was only one way in and one way out of a canyon, but I was wrong. Canyons are long, steep valleys that have multiple entry points and exits. You can enter any way you want, but once you're in the canyon, there is something about its magical properties that makes you want to explore every part in detail and forge a new path.

I've heard all my life that it's my grandmother's prayers that have helped me, but I think it's deeper than that. It's not just my grandmother's prayers; it's all the ancestors whose wisdom helps me grow, learn, and heal. We all have access to this knowledge if we just listen. And guess what? This book is going to show you how.

The Healing Journey Is Now

I REMEMBER WHEN MY GRANDMOTHER DIED. It was the final straw in what I call the worst year of my life. My college sweetheart broke up with me, then my dad—the man who raised me and not my biolog-

ical father (whom I've never met)—had a midlife crisis and started using cocaine, and finally, I had to leave school. I tried so hard to keep myself together, but my body reacted, and within eight short months, I gained eighty pounds. I'd never had a weight problem before, but my trauma was loud, and my body was protecting me. I was in pain, but I didn't know I was in pain.

Being ignorant of your own pain is futile, because ultimately, something will come up and, often, bring back a memory you chose to forget. But that memory has the power to force you to heal. I get it: Why would you circle back to uncovering your deepest, darkest pains? This is why knowing yourself and healing can be broken down into pieces, giving yourself the time to integrate what you uncover and what you learn about yourself.

When I began my first journey in the canyon, I realized that I needed to know the truth of my story. Before starting my shift at Papyrus Paper, I called my mother and asked, "What happened with you and my birth father? Tell me the truth."

She did, and we cried on the phone. After learning the truth, my guides came back even stronger and ready to communicate with me. Once my guides and I started to build a relationship and I began to channel more, I took another look at my astrological chart with clearer eyes. Since astrology was my first love in the esoteric world, I thought I knew everything there was to know. I was wrong. I had to look at the planets from a different angle, from a healing angle. Once I navigated through that intricate layer, it was as though a veil had been lifted, allowing me to grasp the energies that danced around my life path number. In numerology, a life path number is like a blueprint for your life, offering deep insights into your personality, your life's purpose, and the unique path you're meant to walk. It felt like I was engaging in a sacred dance with the universe, where every step and every moment was guided by an energic rhythm that was always there, but somehow I had never acknowledged it until now.

After I faced myself, both my lack of self-worth and my abandonment issues, I began to understand what energies were at play with my life path number. I learned how to lean in to my natural energy. Once that layer was healed, I then opened myself up to what I had been so afraid of for so long: mediumship. I began taking classes and learning how to connect with the other side and building a better relationship with my ancestors. Then, after all that work was done, I knew it was time to create a world that I loved. So I did.

During that time, I learned human design, which blew my mind. Human design fascinates me because it's like a map to the soul's architecture, offering a unique blueprint that guides us to understand our true nature, strengths, and vulnerabilities. It empowers us to navigate life with greater awareness and authenticity, aligning our actions with our innermost being. Human design not only illuminates the path to self-discovery but also fosters a deep connection with the universe, allowing us to embrace our individuality while understanding our place in the larger cosmic tapestry. Human design is not just about self-knowledge; it's a journey toward living in harmony with our higher self. Human design helped me respond to a whole that was difficult to navigate.

And finally I discovered Internal Family Systems (IFS). Internal Family Systems is a powerful therapeutic approach that dives deep into the inner workings of your mind, helping you understand the various "parts" that make up who you are. Think of it as getting to know your internal family. Each part has its own voice, agenda, and role in your life. Some parts may be protective; others might hold pain. And then there's the core self, which is your true essence—compassionate, curious, and wise. When it comes to canyon work, IFS anchors each modality, providing stability and direction as you navigate the deep, dark crevices within yourself. It offers a framework for exploring and integrating the various parts of your psyche, ensuring that, through psychic channeling, astrology, numerology, mediumship, metaphysics, and human design, you remain centered and supported.

This grounding allows for a more transformative journey, helping you face your inner shadows and emerge with greater clarity and wholeness.

But if I hadn't grown through the other embodiment practices, I wouldn't have been able to fully accept parts work. Each phase serves a purpose to deepen our knowledge of self and answer the questions that coincide with each phase. Your intuition grows as you peel back the layers that are blocking you from receiving spirit's call or messages. The modalities covered in this book allow you to see yourself from different angles, and the embodiments will help you develop your psychic abilities. (For additional guided support during your journey, please scan the QR code in the back of this book to access resources for each chapter.)

Trusting the psychic within brings you into your power. It's an act of reclamation. It teaches you to recognize the whispers of spirit and nudges from the unseen realm. It's like you're rebooting your soul's operating system and you're reconnecting to your innate power, a power that many of us have been conditioned to undervalue in a world that often favors capitalistic conquest over spiritual fulfillment. It frees you from seeking things outside yourself and from seeking things you'd concealed within. Just like in *The Wiz*, Dorothy might have been lost, but all along, she had the power within her to get home, and so do you.

And now you will have the tools to use your power. Home isn't just a place; it's a state of embodiment where you're in full alignment with your most authentic self.

As you begin your journey, I want you to think of the questions posed throughout the book as pieces in your ever-evolving puzzle. You are going to grow through this story, through your story, by traveling through your own personal canyon. And all of it is going to come up—all of your trauma, your experiences, your deepest desires. But as you grow through your canyon, you will begin to embody your destiny.

Magic is not just for survival. It's for living a magical motherfucking life. It's time for you to claim your magic in a way that you've never done before—in an embodied way, in a practical way, in a self-assured way. In your past, you have tried to make ends meet or have done things just to get to the next step. But now you have an opportunity to live a life that is full of vigor, that will help you truly step into your truth, your "I AM." That will help you become who you are destined to be.

You will no longer allow your fears to run the show. Your relationships will have the alignment and boundaries needed to reveal your most authentic self. You will be open to intimacy in ways you haven't been before, experiencing deeper connections and true vulnerability. You won't be afraid to go after your dreams, taking chances on what you've been told is impossible. You will silence the voices of those who have dictated what you should be, embracing who you truly are. You'll find the courage to break free from societal expectations and live life on your terms. You will pursue passions that light up your soul, no longer confined by the fear of failure or of judgment. You will stand tall with unshakable clarity and confidence in your purpose, becoming your greatest ally and fiercest advocate.

This isn't a fantasy. It's the reality waiting for you if you dare to step up.

My hope is that, while reading this book and doing the exercises, you will not only answer the questions that are unique to you but you will reflect on the truths revealed. My hope is that you look at these events from a different perspective, one that understands and doesn't blame, one that knows that all things are in alignment for your highest good, whether you can see it or not.

My hope is that the words on these pages lead you toward your truest self.

Our souls came here to do a job, and it's our responsibility to identify and complete the mission. However, the mission can get derailed, at times, by our traumas and our conditioning. As I tell my clients, friends, and family, it might not be your calling to become a voice of truth and do this work full-time, like me, but it is a part of your soul's healing to strengthen your psychic intuitive muscles to bring you closer to source. In this work, not only do we fulfill our soul's mission within this life but we experience the highest level of soul completion in our lifetime.

Healing starts with the parts of you that feel the most broken. Identify what protected you from getting hurt. Address those wounds and say thank you. Forgive the person who you used to be for making the wrong choices in love. Forgive yourself for putting yourself in situations that only faith brought you out of. Forgive yourself for carrying generational emotions that you've never been taught how to shake. The only way you can move forward is through. You *must* make the phone call to speak your peace with your parents. You *must* write a letter to your younger self telling them how much you love them. You *must* pass go and collect what's truly meant for you, but this won't happen until you address what's behind your mental and emotional walls.

Your Magical Motherfucking Download

1. Make a list of things the old version of yourself saved you from experiencing or helped you survive.
2. Pick the top three things, and next to each one write a note thanking your old self for protecting you when you needed protection.
3. Write down what you learned from these experiences, and describe how they contributed to your growth and healing—or to who you are today.

Joy is yours for the taking.
Happiness is yours for the taking.
Thriving in your fullness
is yours for the taking.
Forgive.
Say thank you.
Never look back.
Welcome to the canyon.

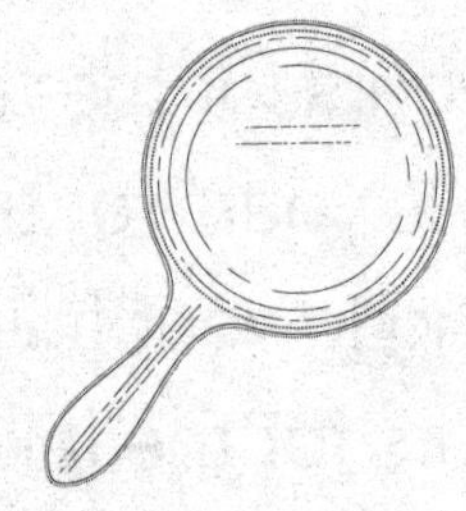

Who Am I?

1

KNOWING YOUR STORY

The Embodiment of Validation

I REMEMBER IT JUST LIKE IT was yesterday. I was eleven turning twelve. My mother and I had just moved into an apartment in Atlanta, Georgia. My parents (my mom and the man who raised me, who I call my dad, though he is not my biological father) had separated a few months back. At first, my mom and I had been living with my aunt in Decatur. My mom is the youngest of eight, and the constant clashing in her family was very harmful to my nervous system. I went from one unsafe environment to another, from my mom and dad fighting each other both verbally and physically to my mom and aunt doing the same. Finally, my mom was able to find us an apartment of our own. Not long after we moved in, a family friend came over. He sat me on his lap and started telling me a story about my parents.

The man said, "You know, Harold is not your father."

I looked at him with very confused eyes. Though spirit had caught my attention on the topic, I had never been given confirmation. But I somehow knew this man's intentions weren't to tell me the truth.

As I continued to sit on his lap, unaware of what he was trying to do to me, he shared that Money (a nickname they called my biological father back in the day) was my father. I didn't know who he was speaking about, but he proceeded to tell me that my mother and this man Money were high school sweethearts and that after my mom became pregnant, this other man didn't want me. He didn't want to be in my life. Later, my mother met the man I knew as my dad. In that moment, this older man, who was trying to take advantage of me, snapped me out of the daze his manipulation had trapped me in.

I started to cry, and at that point he didn't proceed with what he might've had in mind. That information, one of the hardest truths I would ever have to hear, saved me.

Over the years, I did my best to suppress this memory because in my mind it wasn't as bad as other people's stories of abuse. I locked the memory away in little pockets of my brain and attempted to cover it up with feelings of accomplishment and external self-worth. It worked for many years, but as the saying goes, "the darkness always comes to light." I found myself entering my own canyons over and over and over again, relying on performative self-care and self-healing just to survive. I was professing a healing journey all the while secretly harboring unresolved pain. Instead, I was showing up unchanged, reacting with the same old patterns, and failing to develop true emotional intelligence or self-awareness. I thought I was "doing the work," but I could not quite understand that in order for me to discover the treasures of that work, I had to dig below the surface.

But it was the first time I recall raising a wound-shaped question that I would ask myself for many years: *Who am I?*

I remember that night asking my mother if it was true. She replied, "Who told you that information?" After I told my mother what happened, she confessed that it was true. I never told her how the family friend made me feel, but she could tell by the look on my face that he had made me uncomfortable. She must have known there were risks with this man.

A few years later, I recall her telling another family friend that he was like this. It wasn't until I was deeply struggling in my own canyon that I questioned why she had ever left me alone with him in the first place. Communities often skate around the real issues at hand to protect the lies and dysfunction lying underneath. My dad's mother never really liked my mom. When they met, I was seven months old. He fell in love with my mother and me. My mother told me that they had planned to tell me when I was older, in my teens.

I was devastated. All night, I cried at the top of my lungs.

Unfortunately, in most families, and in Black and Brown communities especially, holding secrets is normal. Parents will go to their graves with secrets and use the excuse that it's a form of protection for the child, when in fact it hurts the child and causes more damage. When my mother confessed, I felt like my entire life had been a lie. At that moment, I began to hold shame and confusion in my body, blocking me from my spiritual channels and distancing me from the truth.

For some reason, my eleven-year-old self made sure that she didn't tell my dad that I knew. I wanted the secret to stay between Mom and me, becoming a coconspirator in my own pain and making me question my self-worth. And that decision hurt me more than I could have ever imagined. After that I felt very silent. I went into hermit mode and never really felt innocent again. It was as if my childhood had been stripped away, and I was truly alone in the world. These were the questions I felt but didn't know how to ask:

Why wouldn't someone want me?

Why wouldn't someone want to raise me and care for me?

Why wouldn't someone want to love me?

And ultimately, with the knowledge of my past and how I came to be, who *am* I?

"Who *am* I?"—the embodiment of validation—starts with your story. Our origin stories are the key to our truth and empowerment, setting the stage for how we choose to transform in this lifetime. We all are souls that come here with a mission, and fortunately, we get our assignment at birth, including the parents we are born to, the family we are born into, and the circumstances of our ancestry.

Our souls picked this lifetime. Now is our time to identify the questions that guide our lives. As we validate our origin stories, they become a compass by which we identify and navigate our existence. As we understand and embrace where we come from, we learn to refine these questions and craft stories that serve as a guide for a dialogue between our souls, our human bodies, and spirit. The beauty of our growth in the canyon lies in the unfolding of our curiosity. With each step forward, we discover new questions, expanding our conversation with spirit and deepening our connection to the fabric of life that binds us all. This journey isn't just about seeking answers; it's about being open and willing to receive the power that the questions themselves hold. By allowing them to inspire you, shape you, and lead you to your soul's purpose, you receive the truth.

Why is this important? You cannot heal what you don't understand. You cannot heal what you don't know. Many of us go through our life without ever seeking the truth. Our parents, the people around us, want to protect us, but our stories are what set us free. The truth is what will allow your soul to heal and learn the lessons that you have come here to learn. We will not blame the people who raised us, but we can acknowledge that, in their own way, they usually did the best that they could. And sometimes, they didn't. Sometimes they fell short. But now it is our responsibility to choose what we will do with this information and understand how our stories can heal us.

It is going to be hard to ask the questions. It can be gut-wrenchingly painful to know the truth about your origin story, your birth story, how you got here, why you got here, what happened, and what didn't happen, but that is the starting point on your path through the canyon.

It's funny how the body remembers—and as a baby psychic, my body knew something was off.

Before you start digging into what your own body remembers, remember this: Be kind not only to your caregivers but also to yourself. What you were thrust into, and what you experienced growing up, is not your fault, but it is a part of who you are. This doesn't have to be who you continue to be. You have autonomy and authority to change. (Don't worry, we're getting to that part.) But for now, be gentle with yourself as you begin to discover where you came from, why you are, and who you are.

The Embodiments

THERE'S A SAYING THAT IT TAKES a village to raise a child, and likewise I believe it takes a village to heal a wound. Wherever you are in your journey, you're healing your inner child—or at least, a version of yourself from the past. You might not want to look back, but I can assure you that if you don't stop where you are and go into your canyon and do the work that you need to heal, the pain is just going to continue to show up, often in the most unexpected ways. And then it becomes harder.

The different channels that we use to heal are essential because healing is not a singular approach. Nothing is ever one straight line. There are twists and turns, and at times you need one thing, and at times you need it all. And these channels can provide for all. When you think about healing, the first thing that may come to mind is therapy, but what if you're not ready for that, or what if you're at a point in your therapy where you need to add a few more approaches? Therapy has saved my life on multiple occasions, providing a sanctuary for me over the years. It's a space where I can bare my struggles and receive unbiased guidance. It's in these moments of vulnerability that I feel my spirit calling out, guiding me toward the healing path I need, whether that's through the structured support of therapy or through pursuing my own inner truth. Because no matter how much therapeutic work I do, I have also always had to come back to my spiritual roots and journey. So why are these channels so important?

It's because these channels are the pathways to embodiment. Before we discuss the embodiments, though, we must understand the canyon.

The canyon is also known as the shadow self. Canyon work is shadow work. It is the courageous endeavor to explore the hidden truths of our being. It's the parts of ourselves that we push away, the parts that we neglected, the parts we deem unworthy in fear of being abandoned. It's about unearthing the aspects of ourselves that have been submerged in darkness, the parts that we are afraid to bring to light because exposing ourselves might lead to heartache instead of healing. The canyon is about embracing our fullness, not having a fight with an unknown person in a dark alley.

It's about recognizing that you are meeting yourself to confront the parts of yourself that you've been hiding from the others and showing those parts the power that lies in a truce between the new you and the old you. The canyon is rooted in the belief that within our shadows lie the seeds of our greatest growth and the transformation of healing.

We know the canyon exists, but we also know that once we travel down there, we don't know what's going to happen, and that's scary. Self-discovery and unpacking the layers of our lives is scary. We have convinced ourselves that the better we acclimate to what we think we should be, the easier it will be to cross over the bridge of performative self-awareness and face the harsh truths about the lies we tell ourselves in the name of healing.

It's about acknowledging when we're merely scratching the surface—reading self-help books but skipping the hard exercises or drowning our pain in the relentless grind of hustle culture. It's jumping from one fleeting relationship to another, seeking temporary comfort without confronting our own reflection. It's blaming others for our struggle, refusing to take responsibility for our own growth. This bridge forces us to confront the facade of progress and demand genuine transformation from within.

We cannot continue to bypass our personal canyons anymore.

As we enter the dark canyon, we must ask ourselves, *Who am I?* Start with the embodiment of validation. We first must know our origin stories and how we got here. You are not just the product of an egg and a sperm, but rather the embodiment of your parents' stories and what they were growing through at the time of your conception and while you were in utero. Validating your story will require you to ask hard questions of yourself and others. Some of these questions may be hard to get answers to because your relationships with your parents are broken or not easy to repair, and some questions you may not want to know the answers to. But this is a task that must be done. It's the first step when you enter the canyon. It's the story that your shadow self is most familiar with because it's the essence of you and what you have been dealing with up until this point. Once you know your story, a few things might come up that can cause anger, and this leads to the second phase of embodiment.

The embodiment of anger wants you to ask yourself, *When was I influenced?* This question isn't just about pinpointing a moment in time; it's about uncovering the layers of influence that have shaped your reactions and emotions. When did you first absorb the anger of others? Was it during childhood, in moments when you were told to suppress your feelings? Was it through relationships where your boundaries were constantly crossed? By identifying these moments, you can begin to understand how external influences have molded your response.

And how we understand that is through psychic channeling. Psychic channeling gets to the root of our anger and allows us to get answers from our higher self, spirit guides, and ancestors. Channeling allows us to get to the facts without emotion, without ego. You can receive the clearest answer possible, whether you like it or not. You may have been taught or have even seen that channeling can be an out-of-body experience, but it's actually a bird's-eye view of the highest good of yourself. Why is this important for you? Because when you start unpacking your personal story and learning who you are, you'll get angry. You'll be mad at everyone who concealed your history. By deeply connecting with our origins, we are inspired to expand our view of ourselves and shift from the personal narratives that define us to embrace a perspective as boundless as the stars themselves, revealing a path paved with a sense of belonging that transcends our present and expands lifetimes after us.

Navigating through anger is like navigating a rap battle. Every emotion is a verse, every thought is a beat, challenging you to vocalize your deepest grievances and seek resolution right on the spot. It's like mastering the art of lyrical combat between your heart and your mind—not to start a war within yourself but to understand the underlying story that moves you beyond conflict. In this process, we learn to transform our anger from a weapon of destruction into a tool for healing and nourishment, one that invites you to channel your energy into a powerful performance that is GOAT-worthy, ultimately laying down a track that leads to inner peace and understanding.

Anger processing is a crucial step toward emotional liberation. When we allow ourselves to truly express our anger, we often experience a profound sense of release. It's not necessarily about finding immediate resolution but rather feeling a weight lift off our shoulders, providing a newfound sense of clarity. Our ancestors and spirit guides play a significant role in this process. When our anger makes it through the channel, it's more than a personal release: It can be cathartic across generations. By confronting and expressing our anger, we honor our ancestors' struggles and pave the way for healing in our lineage. This emotional release reverberates through time, helping us break cycles of suppressed emotions and fostering a deeper connection with our spirit guides.

After you process your anger, it's time to embody self. Embodying self is asking yourself, *Where can I surrender in my life and allow ease?* Astrology is one great path. When we're born, the stars align and give us a blueprint. It shows us what might be important to us, who we might love, the relationships we might have with people, and the careers we might gravitate toward. Astrology provides us with the instructions our souls want to follow in this lifetime. Embodying self is hard because it also means we have to forgive who we used to be and be prepared to leave that person behind in order for the new version to shine. We give ourselves permission to embody the fullness of ourselves and to leave behind that which no longer serves us.

We must embrace the cathartic truth that letting go is not just an act of release but an invitation to embody the entirety of our being.

Astrology offers many ways to get to know yourself. You may have identified with your sun, moon, and rising sign as personality traits. These are also tools to get to the core of your being. Once you learn how to use what's in your natal chart, you then open to a world of possibilities. Astrology gives us the framework for who we are, and our life experiences give us the flavor within those frameworks. When we embody self, we can fulfill our destinies or at least be open to what our destinies bring our way.

Next, we look at the energies that help us stay in alignment with the environment in which our soul wants to flourish. Carl Jung states that depression serves as a somber signal from our deepest self warning us of the disconnection between our soul and our body. Jung, a pioneer who ventured beyond the visible shores of the psyche, wanted us to look at this disconnection as an invitation into our souls. He stated that the depth of our emotions often labeled as depression is not a pit of despair or something to be ashamed of but an invitation for transformation. It's a call from our soul, urging us to realign and rediscover the lost harmony between our innermost essence and our physical existence as human beings. When we seek understanding beyond our roles in society and capitalist structures, it challenges us to embrace our canyons and find within them the luminescent path back to wholeness.

Alignment means that you can surrender to what is and operate at your highest capacity within that alignment. Then you must ask, *What's not aligning in my life?* Numerology connects us into alignment because it gives us a path or theme for surrender to help us embrace what is currently happening in our lives. It makes it easier to understand the energies at play instead of judging them and fighting them. For instance, if you know that the theme of your year is going to be about new beginnings, then you will be more open to allowing newness and won't fight change. This gives you the freedom to connect to the natural cycles of your life.

From there, it's time to embrace what is so we can move forward in our skin with the most authenticity. When we embody truth, we embrace the flow of our lives. We know who we are and where we came from, and we accept the best and worst parts of ourselves. We give ourselves permission to exist in our fullness. The embodiment of truth invites you to ask, *How can I connect to what came before me?* Now that you are deeper into the canyon, you will start to second-guess yourself and start wondering if you're on the right path. I believe that the people who have passed before us have the answers that can help soothe our souls while we are here on earth. Connecting to them can help you along this journey in more ways than one.

Once you've gathered information about who you are, how you were influenced, and what's not aligning, it's time to tackle a big question, perhaps the biggest question of them all: *Why am I choosing this life out of all the possible lives?* This is where embodying choice comes in. This may be the scariest part of inner channeling because now that you've unpacked everything and have a clear distinction between what is and what isn't, you must choose. Embodying choice is hard in human form because your body remembers the trauma, the bad decisions, the unhealthy environments, and the limiting beliefs. It clings to our familiar roles. But choice is the only way forward. This is the only way out of the canyon. We leave something behind to make room to grow. We choose our path toward the light by understanding our soul's purpose.

You can stay in the canyon for as long as you want, rehashing stories, making peace with the past, forgiving yourself, and integrating the things you learn about yourself and the world. There's no pressure to be quick. This is an invitation to luxuriate in this slowness of healing. The canyon invites you to be gentle and to be a participant in your unfolding, whether it be physical, mental, emotional, or spiritual. Slowness is not just a pace but a sacred space you cultivate between the noise of your external world and the whispers of what your soul is calling you to caress. It's an invitation to be present with yourself in ways that might feel uncomfortable. This teaches you to accept the ebbs and flows of healing without judgment.

But it's almost time to choose which exit we're approaching. This is where metaphysics comes in. Metaphysics invites you into a realm that transcends the physical. It's a space where the foundational questions of your existence and your reality are being explored. This exploration is deeply spiritual, and it challenges you to look beyond the tangible. It asks you to question things science can't explain.

Once you exit the canyon, you will now be able to take full responsibility for your life. It's time to trust spirit but, most important, to trust yourself. Metaphysics makes us become unwavering in our desires. Choice doesn't say compromise. It asks what you really want and desire. It creates focus.

From the outside, it might look like you can move through these embodiments separately, but this is why we often get stuck on our paths to healing. When my guides sent me the embodiments, I was a bit confused about how they all fit together. But then I reminisced on my journey from baby psychic to your voice of truth, and I realized that having to face the truth of my past through these questions, embodiments, and modalities not only helped me heal but also helped me make peace with my truth and set me on my true course.

Now that you've learned the who, what, why, and when, it's time to walk over the bridge and experience the how. This bridge is no shortcut. It's a rite of passage that is built on patience and wisdom, and every plank is built from lessons of the past. This bridge demands respect, for it embodies the fullness of your experiences. The question now becomes, *How do I want to change my world and the world around me?* The embodiment of change uses human design to help you find your alignment with who you are and stay the course without forcing anything. Human design provides you with a set of your own tools to change yourself and the world around you. It makes walking over the bridge much easier.

The embodiment of destiny taps into the core of who you are through the concept of "I AM." It guides you to fully embrace your purpose by recognizing and integrating the parts of yourself shaped by your experiences. Parts work within Internal Family Systems plays a key role, helping you align these internal dynamics with your higher purpose. This embodiment allows you to step confidently into your destiny, knowing that every aspect of your being is working in harmony toward your true calling.

As I mentioned previously, for additional guided support during your journey, please scan this QR code to access resources for each chapter:

Our Stories Deserve Validation

VALIDATION IS THE ACTION OF CHECKING or proving the accuracy of something. It can be challenging for many of us to connect to our stories. We tend to ignore our trauma. We tend to say it was part of the past—or we replace the messy truth with a more charming story. But our trauma is not only ongoing, living in our current experience; it's also intergenerational and ancestral. Our trauma travels from person to person, from lifetime to lifetime, until one of us decides to heal it. Our stories deserve validation because they are the facts that make up those lifetimes.

They are bigger than just us, and if we are not acknowledging them, we deny the truth. In most cases, but not all, it can be difficult to connect to our stories because there might be instances where we don't have the validation we need to express our truth. When we ignore our trauma, we try to leave it in the past. But when you try to keep things in the dark for a long time, eventually they come to light. Our trauma gets buried both generationally and ancestrally.

Each generation carries unresolved traumas and secrets from the past. These are hidden pains and unspoken truths that were buried by our ancestors. When new traumas occur, they layer on top of old ones, creating a deeper, more complex web of emotional wounds within families. It's like building sediment in the ocean: Over time, each layer adds weight, making it harder to unearth and heal the original pain. This is why it's so crucial to address and process these buried emotions—to break the cycle and bring light to the darkness that's been passed down.

We honor our stories with validation in order to release the pain in our bodies once and for all. After bravely revealing my past trauma, I've heard my mother say, "It wasn't that bad" or "It didn't happen that way." I've had people in my life try to gaslight my experiences and how I felt about them. My healing journey started with simply validating my own experience, allowing myself to tell my own story, regardless of others' reluctance to believe it or to find a shared truth. The truth is, I grew up in a household filled with emotional and verbal abuse. My mother had me walking on eggshells, constantly second-guessing myself and my worth. I internalized this chaos, believing that something was inherently wrong with me. Desperate for answers and a way out, I picked up my first self-help book at the age of fourteen. The book was *Live Your Dreams* by Les Brown. This book became a lifeline, offering glimpses of hope and a path toward healing. It was the beginning of my journey to understand and break free from the patterns of trauma that had been etched into my being.

Through these early steps, I started to realize that the problem wasn't me—it was the environment I was in. To embrace that truth is a sacred act of self-assertion. It's a declaration that my voice matters, that my experiences hold value, and that my human existence contributes to the richness of my world and the world around me.

Life coach Rhonda Britten hosted a reality TV show called *Starting Over*, which gathered women from all walks of life to live together for several weeks. All the women on the show were in a place where they wanted to start over, whether from a divorce or death, from childhood trauma or bad relationships with their parents.

Rhonda had a saying that has always stuck with me, especially when it comes to validating our past. She would ask, "Are you making it up, or is it true?" And in many cases, it is my belief that we take other people's versions of our life as our own. Often, we are not the ones making it up, but we continue to believe the lie because the lie is easier. It's less messy, and it means that we don't have to hold other people—or ourselves—accountable for the choices or actions that were made in the past. We think, maybe it wasn't as bad as I thought, or it's not as bad as it seems, or that's just the way it is. But when we actually learn and excavate the facts, we can see the past for what it was. We can know the truth, and then we can begin to acknowledge and validate our experiences.

We can retire the family lore. Letting go of the narratives others have told me was the most daunting challenge. However, I found liberation in setting aside the tales that were given to me as a form of protection. I had to create safety for myself by releasing these tales, and then I could find freedom.

In the world, our stories matter. And it is our job to validate them—to tell the truth.

Now the facts may not be rainbows and sprinkles and the fairy tale that we would like to perceive them as, but once we acknowledge and validate our experience, we can connect with our trauma—ancestral, experienced, racialized, and ongoing—by allowing our bodies and souls to process that information and to provide us the safety of the truth. From my own healing journey, I realized that because I would skate around the facts, it was hard for me to connect to my trauma. It was hard for me to truly understand my own story. My trauma became an evil twin that I did not want to acknowledge, speak to, or even believe existed.

Instead, I allowed my trauma to become an archnemesis, to become the person who bullied me. Instead of addressing my experiences head-on, instead of knowing my story and asking the right questions, I hid from who I was.

One day, when I was well into adulthood, my mother came back from a funeral where she saw my birth father. After she told me, I asked why she didn't take a picture of him.

I had never seen a picture of him in my life. The funny thing is, when I was growing up, there would always be whispers around holiday gatherings at my grandmother's house. My grandmother was a matriarch, raising several generations in our Queens neighborhood. I remember that during one of the holidays, one of my mom's friends whispered to my grandmother, "She looks just like him."

When you acknowledge and validate your experience, you're able to look at your trauma through clear and factual eyes. That doesn't mean that it hurts less or that you get over it quicker. It just means that you can process it in a way that is conducive for your healing.

To curate the life destinies we deserve, we must know the truth. When we try to fight against the truth, we are fighting against our soul's evolution. The lessons you come here to learn are lessons that help you flow through your life and serve as a backbone to your character; the lessons shape you. When you choose to ignore the trauma and emotional pain that you've endured, you are saying to your soul, *I don't want to evolve. I don't wish to grow.* That hinders your experience here.

Navigating the delicate balance between honoring your truth and maintaining familial bonds can indeed be complex. Embracing your authenticity might place you at a crossroads with those you hold dear, potentially leading to feelings of alienation. Yet if you're not fully aligned with your own truth, it begs the question: How deeply can you really connect with anyone else?

The journey toward living your truth may create temporary distance or misunderstanding with family, but it also opens the door to more meaningful and authentic connection. It's a courageous act to stand in your truth, especially when it might diverge from family narratives or expectations. Being this authentic is the foundation upon which genuine connections are built, with ourselves and with those around us. Once you are able to come to terms with the things that have happened to you, you begin to live with more ease. Imagine a world where the healing we initiate today ripples through time, mending the wounds of our ancestors and laying a foundation of authenticity and love for future generations. This is the vision of intergenerational healing, one where our courage to confront and heal our pain paves the way for a brighter, more harmonious future for all who come after us.

Knowing my birth story validated my experience and gave me a starting point for how to heal myself as an adult, allowing me to forgive my mother and father and take full responsibility for my life. But it also offered me the first connection to the time before my birth, as I began to see the story that extended far beyond my parents' meeting and into the centuries of ancestors who came together before them.

Your Magical Motherfucking Download

We learn specific lessons from the people who brought us here, and in this download, we begin to fully understand what our stories tell and teach us.

- Mother: What your mother went through while you were in utero is what you internalize.
- Father: How your father treated her while you were in utero is what you will express or chase throughout your life.
- You: You will heal the wounds in this lifetime, or you will repeat them in the next lifetime.

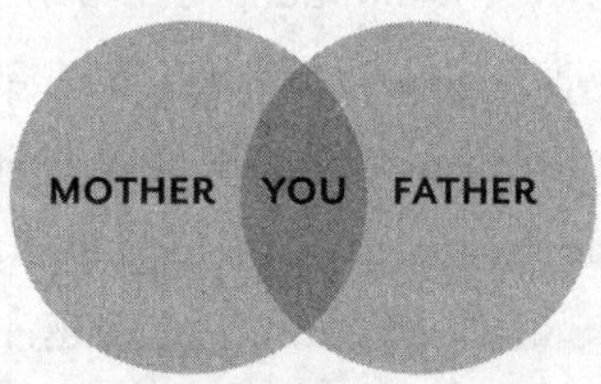

To start, grab a pen, a piece of paper, and a timer. First, sit with your eyes closed and visualize yourself as a baby in your mother's womb. Try to feel into the emotions of what your mother might have been feeling. Try to feel into everything that was happening to you.

After you do that, open your eyes. Write down everything that you can possibly remember about your birth story, including everything you've been told by either of your parents, another family member, or anyone who has told you facts or stories about your birth.

Write down every single experience related to your birth story. What was your mother going through? What was she doing in her life? Were she and your father together at the time? Write down everything that you can possibly think of.

Then I want you to create a timeline. Start from before you were

created, then during your creation, and after. This timeline is going to serve as the beginning of your map through the canyon. The beginning of your parents' story—whether they were in love or not, how they felt about each other, what they were going through while you were in utero—is more important than you think because you were internalizing that experience the whole time. How your father treated your pregnant mother is what you will express or chase throughout your life. And these are the wounds you will heal in this lifetime or that you will repeat in the next one. So, it is your responsibility to get to the truth. It is worth the awkward phone calls. Rock the boat and be bold in your ask. Don't shrink yourself when your mother or father get a slight case of amnesia. Ask them the emotional questions. The wounds you experienced in utero will be yours to heal in this lifetime.

When we confront our pain, we create a ripple effect of healing. It's not just about us; it's about breaking the cycle for future generations. We can offer strength and clarity to our past, present, and future lineage by addressing our wounds today. Our ancestors' struggles don't have to be our legacy. By boldly asking these questions, we reclaim our power and pave the way for a future grounded with resilience and emotional freedom.

This journey isn't easy, but it's necessary. By daring to heal, we honor our past and cultivate a legacy of courage and wholeness for those who will follow. You deserve to know the truth.

Some questions to ponder as you start this work:

- Does my birth story make sense?
- What doesn't feel good about this story?
- Who can I ask about the truth?
- Does this make me feel compassion for my parents?

- Does this make me feel anger?
- Beyond compassion and anger, how does this make me feel?
- What is the story I've been telling myself?
- How has this affected me?

If there are holes in this story based off your memory, it's time for you to do some work. You must ask the people who were there. If you don't have a relationship with your parents, that's okay. This is about fact-finding in the best ways that you can—maybe you have a trusted cousin or an aunt or parental figure who knows the truth of your birth story. Whoever it is, ask them with an open heart. Tell them how much you need to know the truth.

If you have absolutely no way of getting answers from your biological family, or if it's not healthy for you to engage with them, don't worry. We will address this in the next chapter.

Some questions you might ask your family and community as you learn the truth of your origins:

- What was your life like before I was born?
- Do you remember what emotions you were feeling back then?
- How did you feel when you found out you were pregnant with me?
- Were you in love when I was conceived?
- Was it an easy birth? Do you remember any details from that day?

Once you have the story of your creation, this will set the tone for your work throughout the rest of this book.

It's Time to Embody Your Truth

IMAGINE HEALING AND HITTING MILESTONES MENTALLY, psychically, emotionally, and financially and then—boom!—being forced into another canyon when you think you are living your best life. Well, that's what happened to me.

I was on a high. I had moved to a new city, I had healed from some intense trauma, I was in the process of fulfilling my dream to be signed to a major publishing company, and I thought I had met the man of my dreams. Then it all came crashing down in one month. I was starting to write my book when I got ghosted by the guy I thought I was falling in love with. Then, when I announced my exciting publishing deal (for the book you are now reading!), people I thought would be happy for me weren't, and something that was supposed to be so exciting turned into something terrifying. A book? I had to write a book? And with a broken heart?

For the first two months, I was writing through tears and rumination, falling into a depression when it felt like I should have been living my best life. I tried everything to get myself out of my slump, and then I couldn't try anymore by myself. I had to get help. And that's when Lexapro flew in to save the day. Now, before you think to yourself, *I thought it was bad for psychics and mediums to be on antidepressants*, know this: We are all human. Just because some of us have a connection with the divine doesn't mean we're immortal. If anything, the medication stopped the ruminating voices in my head and strengthened my connection to spirit. Only your medical professionals can help you decide what is best for you, but in retrospect, I'm so grateful I trusted my intuition and accepted support when I needed it.

Once the Lexapro kicked in, I was clearer than ever and back into my flow, but that didn't mean I could ignore the canyon that brought me there. I had to look at all the pieces that had turned a lifelong dream into a living nightmare: losing the expectation of love and romance, facing my biggest fears as a Black woman writing her first book, not receiving the support and praise that I thought some of my friends and associates would offer. I had to realize that it didn't matter what those voices were saying inside my head; stronger voices inside my soul—my ancestors and guides—were offering me a different story, as long as I was willing to quiet down the doubt and begin to embody the magic.

Now that we've validated our story, we can look in the mirror and embrace our truth, no matter how ugly or hard it might be. We get the opportunity to see the value and beauty within our stories, and especially our past. To embody validation means being completely honest with yourself, telling and embracing the truth about your existence, no matter what. What is, is.

Our experiences are valid, and the sooner we see the value in our stories, the easier it is to change the channel or the direction of our life, and the more open we are to connecting into a past that can guide us, rather than haunt us.

When you connect to your own voice of truth, you are saying to god/spirit/source,

> I am ready to take complete responsibility for my life.
>
> I am willing to forgive the people who have hurt me in the past.
>
> I am ready to learn from my experiences and move toward a life that is meaningful to who I am and who I am becoming.

When we see the value in our stories, we change the direction of our lives. When we are open to connecting with our past, it no longer controls us but guides us toward thriving in our lives.

I was so afraid of telling my truth because I didn't want to be rejected. I lived a long time with secrets trapped in my body, and it began to show. For years, my family presented a picture-perfect image: upper-middle-class, college-educated parents; a driveway full of luxury cars. But this facade, built on socioeconomic achievements, masked a truth that fueled the chaos within our home. The love, the food, the very energy of our house was laced with lies. It's no wonder, then, that internally, emotionally, and physically, I was living in a constant state of chaos. I had to grow up very fast.

Embracing my truth helped free me, and it helped me root myself in my reality. Once I learned to embody my truth, it gave me permission to release the shame I lived with. It allowed me to remove a layer that was holding me back, which allowed me to get closer to the voice of truth that lived inside me. Embodying your truth is the first step to embodying your destiny. It's hard to know where you're going unless you know who you are and where you've been. This is challenging because truly knowing who you are means that you can no longer deny parts of yourself that you've buried or tried to forget.

It means that you can begin to fully accept yourself.

But to do that, you must get real. You must rip off the Band-Aid, look yourself in the eyes, and say, *This is who I am. This is what I've been through*. Because, quite frankly, anything outside of you is just a reflection of who you feel and believe you are. Once you embrace your story—the real truth of who you are and how you were brought here—the magic begins to happen. Once we understand how our past—our familial and ancestral stories and even traumas—created the life we are now living, our destinies become clearer. They begin to unfold like the melody of your favorite song.

I used to think that destiny was just a means of survival. It wasn't about my spirit or the magic within me; it was about making it through the day, the month, the year. But the more I healed myself, the more my destiny began to sparkle like a crystal. Suddenly, going through the canyon didn't feel like a cold and suffocating experience; it began to feel like magic. And it became a lot easier. The thing was, I was not used to ease. I was used to fighting for my fucking life. Making everything hard. Feeling as though I had to go through something awful to get to the goodness of life. But it does not have to be that way. I promise.

Yes, with the truth came more hurt. I had so many false starts. And at the beginning, I started down the canyon without a map, without clear direction, like so many of us do. But this is why it is so important to embody our truth, to begin this work by acknowledging and validating our stories and lived and inherited experience. We need to work with real answers as best we can—not because we're trying to create more pain but because truth heals.

Embodying your truth is the only way you get to claim your destiny. It's the only way you get to say, *This is who I am*.

Magic Follows Truth

EACH TIME I FIND MYSELF BACK in the canyon, especially after a breakup, I remind myself that I've been here before. I carry the map from my past trips, etched with the lessons and strength I've gained along the way. This familiarity breeds confidence, and I trust the journey more each time. I know that navigating these depths is part of my growth, and with every step, I reclaim my power and wisdom.

Embody Your Magic

Once we understand who we are at our core, we get the opportunity to choose to become something different. The greatest gift we can give ourselves is perspective.

Survival is the state of continuing to live or exist in spite of an incident or difficult circumstance. You should not be living your life "in spite of."

Validating our life story helps us get out of survival mode and tap into the magic within us. Your soul is not "in spite of." Your circumstances, the things that you have been through, may have made you hardened or numb, but it wasn't in spite of obstacles that you survived—it was because of you embodying truth.

When we look at embodying our magic, at embracing our destiny, it shouldn't be for reasons of survival. Our lives are precious, and our souls came here to do a job. Our human experience needs to complete the mission. But not in spite of—not in spite of the pain, the hurt, the trauma—but rather in celebration of those things. When we begin to look at our lives as magical places of existence, we begin to open ourselves up to a world full of possibilities and abundance. If we continue to live our lives from a place of survival, all we will ever know is how to survive. But we can use our stories—even the most traumatic ones—to help us create magic. What if our stories and our pain and our trauma and our experiences were the foundation for building the greatest ritual there ever was? That ritual is our life, and it is here to honor our destiny. What if your pain and your sorrow were the ingredients to build upon a life worth living—not a life in spite of, but in celebration of?

Your truth is part of the ritual. Your pain is part of the ritual. Your trauma is part of the ritual. But it is not the fullness of it. As the truth helps us shift perspective, we learn that everything in our past needed to happen for us to complete who we are becoming, and who we are today is a celebration of everything we have experienced and survived. Validating our life story helps us get out of survival mode and tap into the magic within us.

Look at your life. How magical is it? Are you happy with the level of magic you experience every day? Do you wake up expecting magical experiences and feelings to radiate throughout your body? If not, why not?

When we can see our beginning from different perspectives, we begin to honor our lived experience and the assignment we have chosen. When I validated my own personal story, it led me to a world full of possibilities. Not knowing who my birth father was led me on a quest to figure out who I am. What does that mean to me and for me? I started embracing what I knew was true, embracing the ancestral ties that I could validate. I began to heal the wounded parts of myself by filling in the blanks with information I could control and embrace.

So, maybe I don't know exactly where I get my hips from or my long legs or why I am "a tall short person." Maybe I don't know where my skin tone originates from, or my nose or my eyes or my love of filmmaking, or why I always thought about building my own business and working for myself. But I know that my uniqueness makes me whole. It has allowed me to embody what I know is now my destiny as a spiritual guide and teacher. My not knowing led me to validate the story for others, becoming a voice of truth for their life experiences and destinies. The baby psychic grew up into full-grown adult psychic, and I could see all the magical possibilities in other people's lives.

And then the real magic happened: I began to see it in my own.

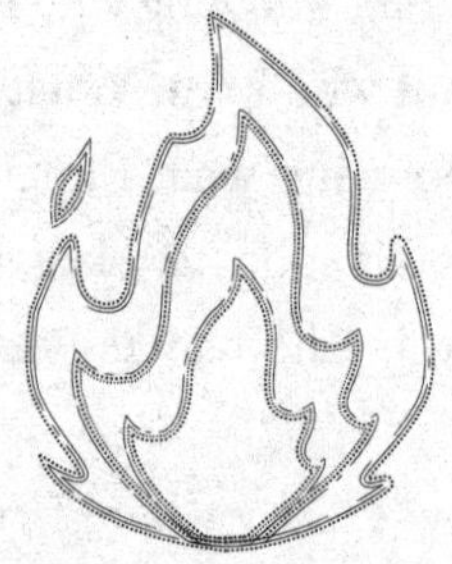

When Did I Get Influenced?

2

PSYCHIC CHANNELING

The Embodiment of Anger

IT WAS A HOT SUMMER Friday in August, about ninety degrees outside and humid, and I had just returned from my coworking space. I was on my way out to get my nails and feet done when I heard a thump at my door. I opened the front door, looked down, and saw a brown box from UPS. I hadn't ordered anything, but at first glance I noticed my guest parking pass poking out of the box. All I could think in that moment was, *He sent my shit in a box?*

I picked up the box as I kept repeating to myself, *He sent my shit in a box?* And then the flood of tears overwhelmed me. I was angry and started to cry. I opened the box and flipped it over. No call, no text, no email. Just a box full of my shit that I had already decided I didn't even want.

Though we had only dated for a few months, I had felt a powerful connection to this person, and he had said he felt the same for me. During our last conversation, he said I was like a storybook, but he needed to take a step back. He said he would call me. He never called me again. Instead, a month after that last conversation, UPS arrived at my door. He had sent my shit in a box.

How could I share energy, emotions, and my spirit with someone who reduced my existence in his life to returning my belongings through UPS—when he lived only seventeen minutes away? As my anger boiled in my body and the tears rolled down my face, I wanted to call him and curse him out, but then I heard a voice. It said, *He doesn't deserve any more of your emotion. You've given enough. You've loved enough. You are enough.*

So, I reached out to my loving community, which consists of my therapist and my friends—even my wise wax lady had loving words for me. That box unlocked a new level in my healing and my connection to spirit. In my anger and pain, I knew that I didn't deserve how I was being treated. I deserved a conversation. I deserved closure. I deserved respect. I didn't deserve to feel discarded and worthless. At first, it felt like every abandonment issue that I thought I had healed up until that point was staring me right in the face. I was back at square one of my healing journey.

How did I get there? How did I get into another situation where I was rejected? Why, when I opened up to someone to give love, was it not returned? I blamed myself. I blamed myself and replayed the relationship down to the detail, which is common for people healing from childhood post-traumatic stress disorder (CPTSD).

What was still in my body that allowed me to attract someone who would behave this way? I started to feel shame and guilt for loving and for living as my most authentic self. The thought of revealing the shameful truth of my rejections made me want to hide again. It made me regret the decisions I had made up until that point, not because I wasn't proud of who I was but because I still had healing to do on certain parts of me. When I told my therapist what happened, she looked me in the eyes and said, "You are more secure than you think you are. I wish you would believe that."

I was surprised but accepted what she said, as she has seen, over the years, my growth and dedication to my healing. So I took a pause, and in that moment, I knew that there was a lesson for me. It's about giving myself freely to people who not only don't have the capacity to handle me but can't even handle themselves.

I stopped taking accountability for someone else's actions and took accountability instead for my response and my self-blame. Throughout the next few months of tears and reflection, I learned two things. Number one, how people treat you reflects how they feel about *themselves*, not how they feel about you. Number two, people can only meet you on your healing journey as far as they have healed and met themselves. These two truths made me angry and frustrated because I thought that my goodness could rub off on people, especially in a romantic relationship. I thought that my healing and my growth would be seen and embraced because I gave love. The work has taught me the art of loving without restraint, and it has liberated me from the shackles of doubt concerning my intuition.

But as I asked myself these questions, I tapped into my guides and asked them what I was doing wrong, and I heard, *Nothing*. They said I did nothing wrong. They advised me to grieve and know that my love will not go unnoticed in the right hands. They said that I must continue doing my work and healing and that when the time comes, there will be a man who will see all of me in my most authentic self and will cherish and adore me at my soul's core. Anger can take control over us, but when we learn how to use channeling to alchemize our anger, we experience a new level of understanding along our soul's journey.

The embodiment of anger connects you to your higher self through learning how to channel that higher self and your guides. Life is hard, but once we acknowledge how the things that happen to us or contribute to our being are fucked up, the more easily we can create a launching pad for change. To embody anger is to get mad and raise hell about where you are and where you've been—while knowing deep in your soul that you have a right to that anger.

This doesn't excuse the bad shit or the people who angered us, but embodying anger gives us a chance to express our true feelings instead of suppressing them, to relate to our inner child and focus on their needs, not the needs of others who can't meet us where we are.

Anger and Your Higher Self

WHEN I THINK OF ANGER NOW, I think of liberation. I think of being free. And that's because anger connects us to our higher self. Anger forces us to ask the hard questions, which lead to our deep understanding of how we have learned to react to life.

When did we get influenced? When did we get conditioned?

When you begin to grieve your old self or when your old self no longer aligns with who you are or who you're becoming, anger shows up. You start looking in the mirror, and you start questioning: *What happened to me?* When we are faced with having to deal with the things that we have buried for a long time, we can begin the grieving process. But in that pain, we might become unrecognizable.

When I received the UPS box, I was unrecognizable. I had to decide between my old self and my new self. My old self would have called and given him a tongue-lashing. I was angry to my core, but my new self knew a boundary had been crossed. I was being disrespected and treated in an unkind manner. I didn't want to give in to a cycle that I had fought hard to transcend. I remember being in relationships in my twenties and showing up at an ex's job because he wouldn't talk to me; I was so furious because he had no compassion for my feelings. But years later, I had grown, vowing to never repeat that cycle nor allow anyone to bring me down to their low vibration.

I was above that now—not in an *I'm better than anyone* way but an *I've healed more parts of myself and I don't feel the need to engage with someone who hasn't even looked at himself* way. I believe that when we begin to heal, we will be tested, and those tests show up in many ways, disguising themselves as the thing we want most.

The tests on our journey through the canyon can and should make us angry. Anger is good. Anger helps us release and deepen our belief in ourselves. Anger, often misunderstood and unfairly vilified, holds an intrinsic value in our nervous system that is critical for personal growth and self-affirmation. The safety in embodying anger lies in our approach to it, especially when our healing journey has moved us away from revenge and destructive impulses. When we understand anger as a part of our healing, we learn to use it as a constructive catalyst rather than a misdirected outburst. When we give a voice to our anger through creative expression, physical activity, or screaming at the top of our lungs, we allow anger to be heard and don't let it spiral into harm.

Anger allows us to connect to our higher self by making us so frustrated and so annoyed and so displeased with where we are that we start questioning everything. And we begin to demand answers, not just from the world around us, but from the world inside us. We see our needs more clearly and map our desires unclouded by others' expectations of us. As we begin to ask questions of our higher self, we also begin to connect with our spirit guides and with our spirit team.

We begin to walk with them through our past, not only our individual past but also our ancestral journey.

I thought it was normal to live in a beautiful neighborhood in a moderately big house. Everyone's parents had nice cars, including mine. I thought it was normal for my father to get a new BMW every year. I remember when Bobby Brown's song "Don't Be Cruel" came out. He talked about a Mercedes-Benz 560SEC, and there was one in my driveway. Fur coats, Louis Vuitton bags, shopping sprees at the finest stores—I thought that was normal. I thought everyone had that access to material riches.

As I started paying attention and as my guides started leading me to different things in my house, I realized that something was off. I didn't have a name for it at the time, but today my dad would be considered a pioneer, as weed is now legal in many states. Unfortunately for my dad and many of his friends, back then they were considered drug dealers. There were, and still are, hundreds of thousands of Black men and women incarcerated for something that is now praised and has been turned into an industry that enriches lots of white folks.

I'm not quite sure when shipments came in, but I could always smell them in our basement. I knew it was weed because my grandmother would always yell at my parents for having it in the house with me around. The smell was unmistakable to me, like a skunk. There would be full trash bags all around our pool table and bar. Pounds and pounds and pounds. I didn't realize that those big trash bags were what allowed us to live like we did. I thought it was an amazing life, but as I found out, it was a life full of secrecy and danger and heightened anxiety. I had no clue that my childhood not only inspired my psychic abilities but also contributed to my unstable nervous system.

I thought it was normal not to invite friends to your house. I would ask to have parties or gatherings, but we couldn't have them at my house. Instead, we would host them at my grandmother's house, which I now realize was a safe haven not only for me but for many others.

I can recollect chunks of my childhood, and but there are other pieces I have lost. I don't know if I meant to block them out or if I had to block them out to survive. But either way, I was conditioned to think that everyone lived this way: that everyone had access to money and fancy things, and that everyone kept secrets. I grew up in a bubble; it protected me but also didn't allow me to have freedom—or access to the truth. It didn't allow me to really be free as a child.

Imagine waking up one day as an adult and looking at yourself in the mirror and not knowing who the fuck you are. Not knowing how you got to this place. This is one reason why it can be so hard to face truth. Many of us continue to put the mask on every day because it is normal for us. Because it's more comfortable that way. Because we don't know of another way to live. But one day the mask stops fitting, and then we get confused, and that's when we need to tap into something outside of ourselves. Something that can give us answers.

Anger connects us to our higher selves by forcing us to get real. Our higher self knows exactly what we need, want, and desire. It is our ego mind that will do anything to convince the higher self that things are just fine, that things are working out, that this is what you want, or even worse, that this is the life you deserve, even when it isn't the life you want.

But your higher self is on the other side of the mirror, looking at you and saying, *That's not true.* That's when conflict happens, and you become angry.

And when you get mad enough, you will start seeking answers. You will want to know: How did I get here? Why am I like this? Who made me like this? How can I move forward knowing this new information that I have? Because this isn't the life that I thought I wanted. This isn't the relationship I thought I wanted. This isn't the job or the career I thought I wanted. And your higher self looks back at you and says, *Then let's find the one you really deserve.*

But you had to get to where you are and get angry enough to realize that there was another option, that there was a way without the mask. When you go through the canyon and you start to take off the mask, it's almost as if you've never seen what was underneath before. You've never seen the trueness of your heart. You've never seen who you actually are.

And that can make you angry too, angry enough that you decide it's finally time to change.

Inner Channeling for Outer Change

ANGER LEADS US TO OUR SPIRIT GUIDES and ancestors because it asks us two questions: *Is anyone out there listening? And if there is, how do we connect with our spirit guides and ancestors?* That is the gateway that connects us to our spirit team, which is waiting to offer us solutions and direction, comfort, and a sense of security in a strange way. Our spirit guides and ancestors are always watching. They are watching when we are in our joy, in our pain, and in our pleasure.

We tend to think that our spirit guides and ancestors have forgotten about us, especially in hard times or when we get angry at the world around us or within us. But what we need to understand is that our anger connects us to our spirit guides and ancestors. It is a gateway to opening that portal of communication. When we are so distraught or so distressed or so upset about our current circumstances, we have no other choice but to open our minds and our souls and listen. Many people say that prayer is the question that you send to your spirit guides, god, and your ancestors—and meditation is where you get the answers.

Psychic channeling allows us to ask the hard questions and get answers from our higher self, spirit guides, and ancestors. Channeling allows us to get the facts without emotion, without ego. It gives us the ability to hear or receive the clearest answer possible, whether we like it or not. Channeling doesn't make excuses; it elicits the hard truth. And the clearer we make the vessel, the deeper we can go.

When our worlds fall apart, right in front of our faces—whether it's the loss of a relationship, a job, a friendship, or a circumstance—

when something shifts, we get angry because that wasn't the plan. We were supposed to spend our life with that person. We were supposed to climb up the corporate ladder from that position. We were supposed to go on trips with our friends and celebrate momentous occasions in our lives together. But source is there to show us another future.

Psychic channeling is a practice that has roots and origins in various cultures, spiritual traditions, and communities. Psychic channeling involves a person embodying an energy or receiving energy from an external source, like a spiritual guide, ancestor, or higher self. As a psychic channel, I serve as a conduit for the knowledge and wisdom that is beyond the material plane. I tap into my guides.

Influential figures have shaped the public's understanding of channeling. In recent times, Jane Roberts, known for channeling the Seth material, opened doors to deeper spiritual insights that continue to influence modern spirituality. Jane Roberts was one of my favorite twentieth-century channels. Jane was an author and poet who channeled an entity named Seth from the 1960s until her death in 1984. Similarly, Esther Hicks, who channels the collective consciousness known as Abraham, has brought the concept of the law of attraction into mainstream awareness, offering guidance on manifesting and living in alignment with one's desires. Both Roberts and Hicks have significantly impacted how channeling is perceived and practiced in the contemporary world.

Throughout history, channeling has been a profound way to connect with higher realms and gain wisdom. This lineage spans across cultures and ages, from ancient shamans and oracles to modern spiritual guides. Each of us contributes to a vast, interconnected tapestry of spiritual insight and guidance. My main guide's name is M. He channels through me for my clients and for the collective. By channeling M, I am not only continuing this rich tradition but also expanding it, helping others access this transformative knowledge in their own lives.

In ancient Greece, at the Temple of Apollo in Delphi, which was considered the most important shrine in Greece, lived a group of priestesses named Pythias. They would enter a trancelike state and were said to channel the god Apollo, and they became one of the most powerful groups of women in history, naming kings and prophesying doom ("Love of money and nothing else will ruin Sparta"). They were praised and immortalized by poets and thinkers from Aristotle to Euripides to Herodotus to Plato to Ovid.

Shamanism is found across Africa and Asia and within many Indigenous cultures. Shamans go through a long and rigorous initiation, which involves fasting and other processes to become spiritual conduits so that they can channel ancestral spirits in order to help guide and heal.

During the nineteenth century, many people started to emerge as channels, channeling messages for the collectives and groups. Helena Blavatsky, who cofounded the Theosophical Society, channeled with Ascended Masters.

Ascended Masters are believed to be spiritually enlightened beings who have transcended the cycle of reincarnation and achieved a state of higher consciousness. They are considered to have mastered the challenges of the physical realm and achieved spiritual liberation. Ascended Masters appear in various spiritual traditions, and they are known by different names. In some cultures, Jesus Christ, revered in Christianity as the son of god, is seen as an Ascended Master. Buddha (Siddhartha Gautama), the founder of Buddhism, is also known as an Ascended Master.

The Seth Material is a collection of teachings and insights from Jane Roberts, who claimed to channel an entity named Seth. Her

work is considered one of the most well-documented examples of channeling and resulted in the publication of over twenty books. Seth's teachings highlighted and brought to life the concept that you create your own reality.

Channeling is my main form of communicating with my spirit guides and ancestors. Connecting with them on a soul level has changed my life and made me appreciate my gift. When I find myself getting angry at my journey, or the world, it brings me comfort knowing that I can tap into source and that I have a space to ask questions and to find answers.

When we get angry and ask our guides, our ancestors, and our higher self what next steps we should take and how we can respond to circumstances, we give ourselves permission to follow our soul's journey.

There are certain parts of ourselves that we have been denied access to, disconnecting us from our most authentic, truest version of ourselves. And when those parts get angry, channeling can help us realize the truth in those matters.

When we access our most authentic truth, we are able to clear our vessel. But our vessel cannot be clear when anger is in the way. Anger blocks us from so many things: It blocks us from joy, it blocks us from happiness, and it blocks us from peace. The anger that boils in us when we don't know the answers can stop us from seeing the purity that life has to offer. It makes us hold on to trauma and remain in situations that don't serve our highest good.

But if we move through the anger, using it to help us channel spirit, then we can begin to clear the pain and the hurt that block us from our passions. Expressing the anger clears the vessel so we can truly connect to source. We can hear the divine callings of our soul.

Psychic Channeling 101

I STARTED GETTING MESSAGES FROM SPIRIT, from source, when I was very young. I would hear someone talking to me, and I was very cognizant that it wasn't coming from the people around me; it was coming from some distant place inside of me. Though channeling and other psychic abilities have been linked to certain mental illnesses, I knew that it wasn't psychosis or anything of that nature. I knew the voices were real, benevolent, and a gift, even when I wasn't always sure it was a gift that I wanted. The ability to connect to the spirit world has a long history of being weaponized against psychics.

I knew that those voices weren't of myself, and I didn't fear them. That's when I started asking questions of the people around me—and that is when the people around me started to get extremely curious as to how I would know things. They wondered also about the questions that I asked, which were always very wise and adultlike, not like the questions of a seven- or eight-year old, and certainly not a five-year-old. I had been called an old soul for as long as I could remember. My grandmother would play songs from the Motown era on her old record player, and I would dance and sing like I had heard those songs before in another lifetime.

My experience with channeling has usually been through hearing a voice or just knowing. Sometimes, a picture will form; other times, a scene will play out in my mind, with voices speaking and telling me something. When my guide M comes through, it's like being in a white room with no doors or windows. And then I hear a voice. It's calm, bold, and clear.

Even to this day, channeling comes in so many ways. When I started channeling professionally, I would have to close my eyes so

I could hear and see. Because my way of channeling is so different and nuanced, when it comes to other people, I take that same approach. But before we get into my methods for channeling, let's dig a little deeper into the ways that many of us access these parts of ourselves, known in the community as the clairs.

The term *clairs* comes from the French word meaning "clear." Combining *clair-* with different senses (like seeing, hearing, and feeling) creates terms like *clairvoyance* (clear seeing), *clairaudience* (clear hearing), and *clairsentience* (clear feeling). The widespread use of *the clairs* to describe these psychic abilities likely emerged in the late twentieth century within spiritualist and New Age circles. But belief in psychic abilities goes back for centuries across many cultures.

In the spiritual realm, the clairs are about having heightened abilities that allow you to tap into different spiritual realms. My psychic channeling has always come in the form of either claircognizance (clear knowing), clairvoyance (clear seeing), or clairaudience (clear hearing). As I channel, my guides and I tell a story that weaves in the past, present, and future in order to help me or my clients move in the right direction.

When I teach others, I explain that there are multiple ways to receive information. But one common method is to notice what happens first. Do you hear first, see first, know first, smell first, etc.?

The clairs offer different ways we can begin to sense the spirit world.

- *Clairvoyance (clear seeing):* When people hear the term *psychic* they often associate it with clairvoyance, which is the ability to see clearly beyond the physical world. Clairvoyance allows you to connect with your guides, ancestors, and other planes of existence

through visions or images. Clear seeing represents the core of psychic abilities that enable you to pierce the veil of the physical world and access deeper truths that you won't normally see. When you embrace your clairvoyant abilities, you open yourself to different realms, where visions and imagery provide a bridge beyond everyday life.

- *Claircognizance (clear knowing):* This is the ability to "just know." It involves receiving intuitive guidance and a deep sense of knowing without any prior knowledge or history about the person or subject in question. Claircognizance can be one of the most challenging clairs to identify and trust because it's often difficult to distinguish between an intuitive thought and your inner voice. Many people possess claircognizance but struggle to rely on it, as it requires setting aside the ego and fully trusting the information that comes through.
- *Clairsentience (clear feeling):* The ability to feel the emotions, energies and physical sensations of others. This intuitive gift allows you to sense the emotional and energetic states that your guides are trying to convey, often through a deep, physical connection. It's like stepping into someone else's experience, feeling their joy, pain, and essence. Clairsentience offers a way to receive insights and messages from your guides, not through words, but through the energetic resonance you feel within your being. When you tune into this deeper frequency, you can connect with the unseen world through the power of feeling. This allows your heart and soul to interpret messages that are sent to you by spirit or the universe.
- *Clairaudience (clear hearing):* This is the ability to hear voices, sounds, or even music that others cannot perceive. These messages can come as external sounds or as an inner voice in your mind, offering guidance from the spiritual realm.

Clairaudience allows you to create a dialogue with your guides, receiving insights and support that can lead to healing. It's like tuning in to a private frequency, where the whispers of the spiritual world provide clarity and direction. This sacred communication offers a profound connection, nourishing your healing journey through sound and voice.

- *Clairalience (clear smelling):* This is the ability to detect odors, perfumes, or other scents that have no physical source. These aromas often carry deeper meaning and can be tied to memories or the presence of spirit guides. For example, one of my spirit guides announces his presence with the scent of cigars, signaling that he is near and ready to communicate. These sensory signals act as a bridge, offering insight and guidance from the spirit realm, reminding you that you're never alone in moments of connection.
- *Clairempathy (clear emotional feeling):* This is often recognized as the hallmark of an empath. It is the ability to directly feel and understand the emotions of another person or spirit. Unlike clairsentience, which involves physical sensations, clairempathy is purely emotional, allowing you to experience the raw, unfiltered waves of someone's else's feelings. Connecting with the emotions of your spirit team through clairempathy helps you deepen your bond with them and yourself, creating an emotional connection that fosters understanding and intimacy on a spiritual level.
- *Clairgustance (clear taste):* This is when you have the ability to psychically detect tastes that aren't physically present. It might manifest as tasting garlic, blood, or experiencing an inexplicably dry mouth. These sensations often occur when a spirit is trying to connect with you or someone else. Through this unique

connection, your taste buds become a tool for receiving a message from the spiritual realm, offering insights and guidance through vivid otherworldly flavors.

- *Clairtangency (clear touching):* This is the ability to receive psychic information through touch. By holding an object, a person with this gift can sense its history, the people who have owned it, and even the era of its creation. This unique connection allows them to absorb the object's energy and uncover the stories embedded within it. It's a profound way of connecting to the past, revealing the silent narratives carried by the objects we hold.

As you begin to channel, look for and feel what happens first. To initiate meditation, it's essential to create a serene and sacred space where you feel safe and will be undisturbed. If silence doesn't work for your meditation (it doesn't work for me), you can use music or binaural beats, which are a form of sound wave therapy that can profoundly affect your mental and emotional state. When you listen to a slightly different frequency in each ear, your brain perceives a third frequency, which is the difference between the two. This third frequency, known as the binaural beat, can help synchronize your brain waves, leading to states of deep relaxation, focus, or even heightened creativity. It's like a musical bridge that guides your mind to a desired state, making it a powerful tool for meditation, healing, and personal growth.

Focus on your breath, allowing yourself to become deeply relaxed and open to receiving guidance and direction. Intention is everything in this process.

After you close your eyes, or after you quiet your mind, what happens next? After I meditate, I first get an image, then I hear sounds. However, if my eyes are closed, I hear first, then I see. So, there are so many nuances to channeling. What happens for you?

Do you hear first? Do you see first? Do you feel first? Do you smell first? Do you know first? Do you see shapes, images, or colors in your mind's eye reminding you of someone or something? Do you suddenly smell a loved one's perfume or cologne when there's no physical source for this scent? Or do you suddenly know the answer to your question, like the exact steps to take? Does a song with profound lyrics pop into your head and bring you back to a moment in your life that you can remember vividly? The more you tune in to these senses, the more you may be able to recognize which ones are dominant for you. Keep an open mind and take note of what you are experiencing.

Some people get chills or other sensations in their body. Whatever happens first, the response is quick. Some people just know instantly. It is an experience that comes from source, from spirit, and through you. Trust it. Once we understand what happens first for us, then we build on that skill, strengthening our connection to source, to spirit, to our ancestors, and to our guides.

The most common clairs are, of course, clairvoyance and clairaudience. When you say *I'm psychic,* or when you have psychic abilities or intuitive abilities, the first thing that people are going to think of is clairvoyance.

Learning to channel is no different than learning a new language. We begin to practice, figuring out the best ways to learn, to begin to communicate, to translate the messages, and to understand their meanings.

When you begin to channel, be willing and open, but also be ready. There have been many times when I wanted to deepen my relationship with source, but I just wasn't ready. Channeling can be very scary because, depending on what you are asking spirit, you might not be able to handle what will be downloaded. You know you are ready when you ask repeatedly. The more you ask, the clearer the answers will come, and the answers will be unbiased.

At first, I wasn't sure if I was connecting, but over time, I became more willing and open. As I practiced and deepened my process, I would ascend to a new level of sensing. I would start having more visions or hearing more voices. People who had passed on started coming to me. The first time I can remember this happening, I was around eight years old. And I had to stop being scared of them. I had to stop seeing this connection as a curse and begin treating it as a gift—and as a strength.

Fear is a natural response as you start opening yourself up to spirit. News flash: Source, your ancestors, god, and your guides have always been right next to you. They are the little voice that is telling you, *Don't go to the store* or *Go back home* or *He's not the one.* That's the spirit realm helping you out, you just might not have been cognizant of the relationship. It is always guiding you, just like mine was guiding me when the UPS box showed up at my door unannounced and a little voice took over in my body. It told me not to call my ex, to take a step back from him, to breathe while I sat and looked at my stuff on my kitchen floor. That voice was helping me even when I wanted to get answers, even when I questioned so much in that moment, including myself. But when I tapped into my guides, I knew that with this box, the way the relationship ended wasn't about me.

Think of the guides like a GPS for the soul, always up-to-date and guiding you in the best direction. It's like having a friend who always knows the best restaurants and hotels and who never leads you astray. The guides don't want to lead us into danger; they are here to support us and help us through our journey, even though we can't see them.

In moments of doubt, I've had to trust my guides and my therapist, no matter how hard it was at the time. You see, when we make a connection to our spiritual team, it takes courage to trust and rely on what they are saying and how they want us to move and be in the world. It takes daily practice. It takes practice to listen and follow instructions. It takes willingness. We need to get to know them.

What I, and many of us, didn't realize was that my connection to source—to my guides, to my ancestors, to spirit, to god—was literally my gateway to helping myself heal. The more my connection strengthened, the easier it was for me to heal. The more resistant I was to my connection and my reliance on source, spirit, and my soul, the harder it was for me to acknowledge the truth and accept life. But the more I strengthened my connection, the more self-aware I became and the more my path through the canyon became clear.

There's a song by rapper Bone Crusher called "Never Scared," and it always reminds me of tapping into the spiritual realm. When you are facing your shadow self through the canyon, it's about facing what's in front of you, not behind you. It's about facing the unfamiliar. And we need not be scared as we face those truths. Trust me, as we build and strengthen our connection to a higher source, we realize that we don't ever need to be scared because we have our spirit team beside us. When we are living a magical life, every step is a sacred dance. Each heartbeat is a connection moving us in harmony with the universe's rhythm.

Your Magical Motherfucking Download

We will use guided meditations to connect with our higher self and allow our guides to come in and give us the answers we seek. You might want to record yourself reading this section so you can relax and follow the instructions.

To start this meditation, you need to be in a quiet place, seated comfortably or lying down.

Relax your mind.

Close your eyes.

Begin to breathe in through your nose and out through your mouth.

Do this at least seven to ten times, enjoying these deep inhalations.

Once you have a regular pattern of breathing, inhaling through your nose and exhaling through your mouth, I want you to visualize a gold ball spinning on the top of your forehead. And as that gold ball spins on the top of your forehead, it starts dripping gold light or gold particles on the top of your head. And with every spin, the gold light fills up your body.

As your body fills with the gold light, it expands throughout your room. Throughout your home. Throughout your neighborhood. Throughout your city. Throughout your state.

And it expands until all you see is a gold light, and you know it extends far beyond your vision.

As that gold light surrounds you and embodies you and all that is all around you—and as you're breathing—call forward spirit source, your guides, your higher self, your ancestors, or whoever you want to call forward.

And ask them a question.

Once you ask the question, pay attention to what happens next. Do you see? Do you hear? Do you taste? Do you feel? Do you know?

Once you have established what happens first, continue the conversation. Ask as many questions as possible. Ask: *Who am I?*

Then listen.

Then ask: *What is the root cause of my anger?*

Then listen. Then ask any other questions you want.

Here are some to consider:

- What lessons am I meant to learn from the anger I'm experiencing?
- How can I release the anger that no longer serves me?
- In what ways can I transform my anger into a positive force in my life?
- What messages or warnings does my anger carry for me?
- What steps can I take to prevent anger from overwhelming me in the future?

Once the conversation is done, grab a pen and a piece of paper and write what you heard, saw, smelled, tasted, knew, felt, or experienced. And that is the start of your relationship with psychic channeling.

Anger Gives Us the Will to Change

IN MY LIFE, I'VE NEVER DRASTICALLY CHANGED who I was or who I wanted to be because I felt happy and cheerful and delightful. It was in my anger, my frustration, or my confusion that I began to ask the hard question: *How did I get here?*

Discovering myself in a place I didn't set my sights on stirred a surge of displeasure within me. That anger fueled the change. That anger pointed me in the right direction. That anger was the gateway from my mind to my higher self. It allowed me to open the doors to my higher self, to channel, to ask the right questions, to be open and willing to receive the truth.

When we express our anger, this starts our journey through the canyon. Our anger gives us the fuel to muster up the courage to push forward with or without the will. *Will* refers to the desire, inclination, or choice of wishing, choosing, or intending to move forward or act toward something. There are many times when you don't have the will or desire to move in a direction that can change your life from where you are to where you want to be. However, anger can give you the will you need to guide you through your canyon.

Canyon work is never easy. Our bodies don't naturally adapt to transformation; they'll need to embrace the new selves we become, in time. Our bodies aren't used to the changes that will take place during our transition from our old self to our new self. There have been many times when I didn't know if I was going to make it through, but I did. There were times when my nervous system was fighting me so hard to just remain the same. Anger triggers the body's fight, flight, or freeze response, which produces adrenaline and cortisol. Holding on to anger isn't good, but when our bodies have been conditioned not to lean in to our anger, *not* leaning in to our anger creates a false sense of safety. Anger is an emotion that we fear. Many of us are taught to suppress our anger to appease those around us, to "keep the peace." When I was growing up, I heard things like "Children are to be seen and not heard." I was taught to respect my elders and not let them know they hurt me, no matter how they might be disrespecting me or my boundaries.

I learned to hold my anger within. I learned to let it boil up and burst out in a wave of emotions. My anger made me turn my back on my most authentic self. Suppressing my anger taught me how to walk on eggshells. When I was frustrated, I would have vivid images of hurting myself or others because I didn't know how to channel my anger in a safe manner to feel seen and heard. Once I learned how to use my anger to connect with my higher self and my guides, I was able to get it out of my body. I was able to let it take control over me and release itself—safely—through my body. Channeling connected me to my emotions. My anger helped me realize I was hurting or unhappy. I couldn't hide it any longer. My anger burst through to help me acknowledge other emotions.

Use your anger as a gateway to connect to your higher self, a gateway to your truth, a gateway to your knowing. When we tap into our anger, we tap into our feelings in a profound way, and our feelings connect us to our destiny.

Our anger is what sends us into the canyon. There are things that will come up that will scare us, things that we have pushed down deep inside that we must heal. Addressing them will free us.

Anger starts us asking questions. *What happened? Why did this person do this to me?* It gives us the wherewithal and the courage to connect deeper, to channel more often, and to hear what spirit is trying to tell us. I'll warn you now, it takes some time to really listen, and it might be painful. You want the things that you want. You want the results that you want. But spirit and your soul know what's best for you; to change, we must trust them. So, as you go through your own personal canyon, you will begin to transmute your anger to heal your trauma.

Psychic channeling is essential to your healing journey because

through your higher self and through those guides that have been with you since the day you were born, protecting and guiding you, you can begin to pinpoint when you were influenced and what happened to you along the way.

After each traumatic event in my life, psychic channeling has proven to be the gateway to learning how to use my talents and gifts in the spiritual realm. Now to some of you that might sound fucked up, but I feel that every trauma, everything that has happened to me has brought me closer to spirit, closer to source, and more in tune with my psychic abilities, more in tune with the spiritual gifts that I hold. I feel that times of struggle are when my guides and spirit connected to me most deeply. My visions became stronger. My foresight and my knowing became clearer.

Many of us were taught to tiptoe around the emotions bubbling inside. This creates an aggressive and sort of violent image of ourselves, causing us to fear our own emotions. But our guides consistently remind us that anger is a creative spark in our lives. Anger shows us that we are not safe. Anger lets us know that we are out of our bodies, and that we are not in control. Anger ignites our feelings, our emotions. It helps us understand how real the situation is that we're dealing with.

Anger helps us acknowledge our emotions and tap into our destiny.

I truly believe that some of my best transformations have come through anger. I've moved. I've left bad relationships. I've set boundaries with unhealthy people. I've changed jobs or passions or hobbies. I went back to school. Anger shows us how things really are and offers us the opportunity to look at ourselves and say, *I am making the choice to receive something better in my life.*

My anger has launched life changes that have been so beautiful.

As you go through your own personal canyon, you will find that

anger is part of the grieving process. It's the process of moving from the old self to the new self.

Anger helps you heal the trauma.

You may have heard that we are all just souls having a human experience. What that truly means is that your soul is trying to infuse your human experience with your purpose and what you have come here to do in this lifetime. It is not always easy.

When you feel pulled in a certain direction—to move to a new state or country, to leave a relationship or job, to go on a trip—what is that force? That is your soul. Listen to your guides. Channeling helps us connect where we are to where our soul knows we should be.

Instructions to Channel Right Now

1. Acknowledge: Close your eyes and take a few deep breaths. Remember a recent situation that sparked anger in you. Allow yourself to feel this anger all throughout your body without judgment or suppression.
2. Deep dive: As you sit with your anger, ask yourself what other emotions are hiding beneath it. Do you sense hurt, fear, disappointment, or perhaps a sense of injustice? Let these emotions surface. Feel each of them.
3. Express: If you're comfortable, express these emotions in the extra space at the end of this box or in your journal. You can write or draw what you are feeling. The goal is to externalize these feelings in a tangible way. If you need to get up and jump up and down or scream at the top of your lungs (this is my favorite method), do what feels good to you.
4. Reflect: After expressing these emotions, take a moment to reflect on the experience. What did you discover about your anger and the

emotions it was masking? Write these discoveries down so you can refer back to them.

5. Release: Conclude this exercise with a few deep breaths. With each exhale, imagine the emotions releasing from your body. With each inhale, envision yourself filling up with peace.
6. Contemplate: In the next few days you might feel underlying emotions moving through your body. Release them.

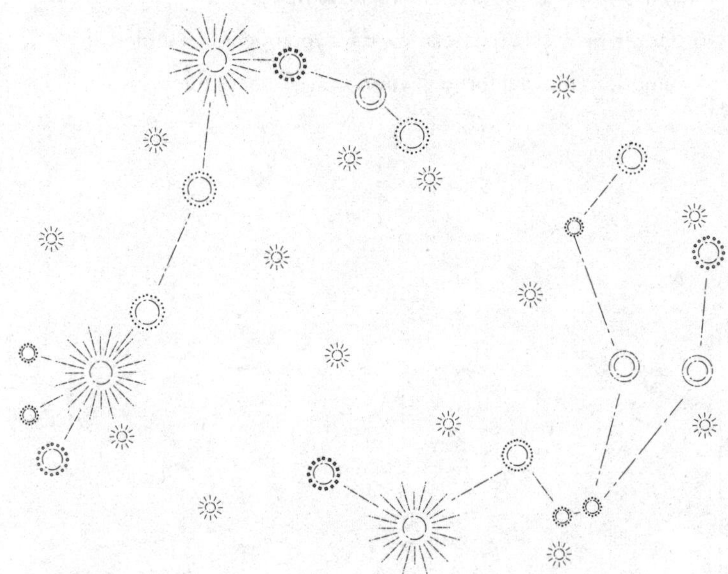

Where Can I Surrender in My Life and Allow Ease?

3

ASTROLOGY

The Embodiment of Self

I ONCE HAD AN ASTROLOGY READING by a man named Ray, who was what I call an old-school astrologer. When we had our session, he looked at me and said, "At the age of four, you had a traumatic event in your life that changed the course of how you see yourself. It left you with scars. But since then, you've been trying to come to an understanding of who you are."

And I knew exactly what he was talking about.

When I was four years old, I spilled a cup of hot tea on my body. By the time my parents had gotten me to the hospital, it had gone from a first-degree burn to a third-degree burn. The severe injury on the left side of my body kept me in the hospital for almost two months. During that time, my parents and other family members would visit during the day, but not once did anyone stay with me overnight.

I have a skin graft on my left arm, left shoulder, and left breast. And because it happened so early in life, I don't remember my body without my burn. I had no clue that experience was trauma. I just thought those were the cards that I had been dealt. But as I got older and as more traumatic events started piling on top of one another, my pain became so unbearable that finally my whole body just shut down. Life simply became too hard.

This massive event left me feeling abandoned and questioning my worthiness, but the more I began to understand my astrology, the more I saw how those wounds were stitched in the stars. Astrology has the power not only to tell you about yourself and how you move in the world, relationships, careers, and community but also to assist you in understanding and accepting the world at large.

As I sit here writing this book, a major transit is occurring with a Venus retrograde in Leo. During this retrograde, relationships are being tested and many breakups have occurred, including my own. But also, long-term celebrity couples are breaking up one after the other, people who folks thought were inseparable are now filing for divorce. This transit is collective, and everyone feels it, as we are asked to reevaluate what matters most in our relationships and what we value in our partnerships, both romantic and platonic. This transit is painful not only for me but for many people around me. If something had been barely working before, during this time it's falling apart—and drastically. It is an unhinged time. Learning how astrology can help us navigate the world, our communities, and ourselves gives me a quiet acceptance that I never knew I needed.

Now don't get me wrong: I don't blame astrological transits for my successes or challenges. But astrology helps me understand the energies at play. You can look back to certain transits that happened and see trends that had the potential to affect not only you but also the collective around you. In 2020, there was a Pluto conjunct Saturn, and I vividly remember speaking with an astrology peer in December 2019 about what would happen. She predicted something major, but we couldn't put our finger on it. All she said was that the world would never be the same after, and a few months later we were in a global pandemic and didn't know what was going to happen—or how we might all be changed. This is astrology at its core. It doesn't necessarily predict exact outcomes, but it offers grounding context and a sense of what might come. It might not be able to predict the outcome of the game, but it can definitely describe the court, the ball, and the rules.

Even with a decade of astrology knowledge, I do my absolute best not to judge each sign. But life has taught me to take it into consideration. When I started dating, it was a free-for-all. I would date someone of any zodiac sign, which taught me a lot. I am a "try it out before I make a final decision" type of woman. However, when I dug deeper into astrology, I discovered that I couldn't date just any zodiac sign. Now before you go into a diatribe about not judging your potential romantic partners just by their signs, I would say that after unsuccessfully dating the same signs with the same underlining characteristics, you begin to realize that some signs are simply a better fit, and some signs can be a very bad fit. It's more of a guiding principle than a strict rule.

Love signs are some of the most popular astrology searches on the internet because a lot of us are trying to find love, and we are seeking guidance to help us find the right partner. Many of us are on a journey, seeking out that one soul who resonates with ours. We need to find areas of connection to guide our search. Astrology helps us surrender to our life and our life path by showing us how the game is played, so we can try to create a better outcome. Instead of comparing to the past, we can name how we want the outcome to be. By clearly envisioning and setting intentions for our desired future, we can direct our energy and actions toward manifesting that reality, aligning ourselves with the universe's guidance and our true purpose.

I have a stellium in my fourth house in my natal chart. A stellium is a place of profound significance where more than three planets gather in one house and sign. It spotlights your strengths, challenges, and soul's lessons. It can help you understand your deepest desires and your true path. A stellium is a call to dive deep and embrace the unique blend of energies that illuminate your mission, your purpose, and your growth. Having a stellium in Pisces in my fourth house means I have intimate spiritual and emotional connections with my ancestral roots. The fourth house is also an anchor to the natal chart, housing the essence of my roots, my home, and my soul's core.

This stellium magnifies my sensitivity toward my family's past; it connects me to my lineage, which highlights my psychic gifts, my emotional depth, and the things I need to heal in this lifetime. It calls for me to be the one who transforms my lineage. When I learned this, it showed me the power of astrology, and it gave me a clearer picture of my place in a family where everyone has siblings except for me.

In surrendering to our astrology placements, we are free to heal on a deeper level and understand how our destinies have been written in the stars since the day we were born. When you are born, your birth time and date create a blueprint that unfolds throughout your life. It's a moving map that changes with transits and progressions of the stars and planets.

My biggest pet peeve is when people say astrology doesn't work,

and when I ask them if they have ever had a reading, they say no. Unlike personality tests like Myers-Briggs (invented in the 1940s) and the Enneagram (in the 1910s), both of which have become extremely popular over the last decade, astrology is ancient and pinpoints exactly what is happening in the stars at every moment in the past, present, and future, including the moment you were born. As you travel through the canyon, the story of your cosmic placements can act as a map, making your journey easier and allowing you to surrender to what you do not know.

To surrender means to yield power, control, or possession of something or someone to another source. Some might say that when you surrender you give up, but I believe that when you surrender you give in. You give in to the grace that spirit/source has for your life, and you can allow ease and flow to happen. When we begin our healing journey, remove our masks, and start to unravel our trauma, we allow spirit/source to bring us the people, situations, and experiences that invite us to heal and evolve into our greatest selves.

Surrendering and allowing ease will be one of the most challenging things we can do in this lifetime. It's because our traumas have allowed us to develop a false sense of control; we feel that if we can control our outcomes, we will be safe. But as many of us have learned the hard way, control does not equal freedom or joy. This way of thinking only interferes with our soul destiny.

Think of a moment when you arranged the pieces of your life's puzzle, aligning each aspect with precision and care, only for an unexpected whirlwind to scatter your plans. I invite you to journey inward and document any emotions that were birthed from disruptions like this. Don't just think about the surface emotions, but reflect on the disappointment and how these moments shaped your very being, identity, and path. Now consider how these experiences honed your intuition, amplifying your sensitivity to the unseen currents in your world and the world around you. Think about how each roadblock and detour not only tested your resilience but also brought you closer to your purpose and destiny. As you write down what comes up, recognize how these plot twists contributed to your progress here on earth. Through this process, recognize the beauty within the chaos.

Knowing your natal chart can show you what you are dealing with and how you can heal with these placements. Even setting aside the energetic elements of astrology, the scientific guidance it offers—what stars and planets were positioned in relationship to Earth during your birth, critical junctures in time and in your personal history, and how you connect (or don't connect) with other signs—gives you the opportunity to make decisions, heal, and thrive using your own blueprint. Astrology can predict the best times to get married, start a business, and many other things, but one of the biggest benefits that it offers us is the ability to dive deeper into our truth. Our soul has picked the situations and circumstances that we will experience in this lifetime, but our free will makes us resistant to the changes that we will grow through.

To surrender is to accept that you don't have control over the outcome. It is to accept that there is a chance that whatever you do or however much effort you put in, you may not get the results you had intended. But what we can control is the energy we put into something and the intention we have. My way of surrendering starts with asking myself if I did my best, because deep down inside, I know I am capable of great things. There are situations on which I can look back and recognize that my best efforts and best intentions did not lead to the desired outcome.

In my romantic relationships, platonic friendships, and business partnerships, I've shown up and given it my all—or at least as much as I could until things fell apart or were out of alignment. In those moments, I've hurt deeply, and the pain brought me back to myself and my canyon to heal deeper, to learn more, and to surrender. We often think of this surrendering process as struggle, but I believe that with the tools we have around us, especially astrology, we can relax through surrender, we can find breath and ease and acceptance. Now, I realize this is especially hard to consider if your primary tool has been control. It was mine too. During this surrendering process, we think it must be hard. To surrender and allow ease offers so much uncertainty that it can be heartbreaking to our human self, but on the other side of surrender is our soul's destiny. Surrendering and allowing ease is our soul's way of giving us permission to work with destiny and not against it. It allows us to alchemize our pain into pleasure and to begin to live the purpose of our existence.

When we surrender and allow ease, we hold space for the parts of ourselves that have been hurt and traumatized. We give a voice to our past and see a brighter future.

The embodiment of self connects you to your emotions and your inner child through astrology. Astrology is our soul's map, helping us solve problems based on transits and progressions, letting us know what's to come using predictive techniques, and giving us the framework for who we are and how we relate to our life experiences.

Astrology as a Path to Self

ASTROLOGY GIVES US A MAP THAT allows us to alchemize our past, engage with our present, and plan for our future. When I started my healing journey in my early twenties, my astrology studies took a turn for the best. I experienced a lot of loss in one year. My grandmother—the woman who helped me hone my gifts and step into my spiritual self—died. My college sweetheart broke up with me. My relationship with my father was strained due to him having a midlife crisis and coping with it through narcotics. I felt lost, as if my life were falling apart. And yet, it was this very same year my psychic abilities also became stronger.

As I began to study the astrology of that moment, I saw that I had heavy fourth house placements. The fourth house symbolizes home, family, and the mother figure. It also represents ancestry, our foundation, and how we plant ourselves. The fourth house is also the home within ourselves and the place we create to be our own personal sacred sanctuary. Understanding how my fourth house played such a heavy role in what I was growing through at the time helped me start therapy and get the help I needed when I was at the darkest place of my life.

Astrology has given me the freedom to know what I am working with when it comes to my own healing journey. Healing is not linear, and when you use astrology as a path to yourself, you gain a better understanding of how it helps you face the challenges that are occurring in that moment, offering a framework of perspective outside of your own actions.

Like any other modality, astrology is an energy we exist in. It provides us tools to explain what is going to happen and why—and when—it might happen. Astrology provides the right environment for those energies to communicate with us—and to flourish. If you look at astrology as an environment instead of a physical place or thing, you can start to appreciate what it offers you at any given time in your life. Astrology is expansive and can offers tools to learn, grow, and heal. When we are in the dark parts of our canyon, as I was the year my grandmother died, astrology illuminates a journey to surrender and accept who we are by seeing our truth within various aspects. It helps us see the archetypes of our mother, father, family, and potential events.

Any true astrologer should be able to look at your chart and identify the significant events in your life. And I find anyone who has a real reading walks away a believer. This is because astrology leaves clues. This doesn't have anything to do with years and years of experience. It's about how the astrologer can translate your chart, highlighting your unique story through their lens.

It is my belief that anything works if you allow it to work. Now whether that thing works to your current vantage point or perspective is one thing, but astrology is about giving you the answers you need to hear, not the ones you want to hear.

The tools astrology offers work. It gives you permission and a path to surrender and accept who you are. Many people look at just their sun sign and then claim, "That isn't me. Astrology doesn't work." But your sun sign is a very basic and egoic part of you and your personality and upbringing. Your sun sign is like that foundation on which your house is built. In the canyon, referring to the stars can teach us to surrender to the environment we are in at any given time. It allows us to accept who we are and what we are working with to release personal responsibility for things we can't control. It enables us to embrace our true selves and the circumstances we're dealing with, freeing us from the burden of blaming ourselves for every minor detail.

Some people don't trust astrology because the cards that they have been dealt seem to contradict their sign. I can have the same placements in my chart that many millionaires have, but if the way I was raised and the environment I lived in didn't offer that path to me, how can I trust that it truly works? I can't. And it will be a challenge for me to gain self-acceptance through this tool. A more pragmatic approach is using astrology to help me rectify my past, surrender to my present, and have more control over my future.

Astrology for me has been a gateway to the possibilities of my life. I'm not just a dreamy Pisces who is out of touch with reality. I am a Pisces who has had to use my Neptunian disposition to survive the realities of my childhood. My Pisces sense birthed my psychic abilities, but it also allowed my imagination to wander far from the reality of the external trauma and environment I grew up in. Astrology allowed me to see the past, understand my present, and embrace the possibilities of my future.

I like to say astrology found me in my teens, when I felt the most isolated. I thought different and felt different. I knew that life had something bigger to offer me, but I couldn't pinpoint what it was. I went to Barnes & Noble and found *The Only Astrology Book You'll Ever Need* by Joanna Martine Woolfolk, and my mind was blown. I felt like the book was calling me. The cover was a deep purple—which at the time was my favorite color—and I went home and devoured it. It showed me so much. It even confirmed why my first love and I were so compatible. His sun sign was my descendent. (Your descendent is the opposite of your rising sign, which rules your seventh house.) It showed me my career possibilities as well as some of the challenges I began facing during high school within my family structure.

Astrology has taught me how to see the possibilities of who I could be rather than just what was presented to me. As I began to do my healing work, I was able to use the tools of astrology to help fill in the missing details of my own life, mapping the traumas and triumphs in my chart. I began to understand why things happened and why I did things, and the chart offered me my life's design.

Start by familiarizing yourself with your birth chart; it's like your personal cosmic blueprint. Understanding the placements of sun, moon, and rising signs will give you a solid foundation. From there, explore how the planets interact with these signs and houses to see how they influence different areas of life.

Now I want you to know that astrology doesn't excuse the bad behavior of people who have harmed you along your journey. But it can give you a perspective on why things happened the way they did. As you explore this question of surrendering and allowing ease in your life through the lens of astrology, I want you to imagine having the information to help yourself heal now. Astrology offers us a unique blend of the diverse aspects of our identity within those frameworks, granting us permission to explore levels of ourselves that society won't allow us to, the parts conditioning takes away from us. Astrology acts as a gateway, not just to the present moment, but to the echoes of our past and the potential of our future. Astrology gives us the permission we often don't find in our daily lives to explore the depths of our being.

Your Magical Motherfucking Download

Astrology gives us the tools to forge a greater path and purpose within our life because the answers are already there. Yes, we have free will, but that free will is limited to an environment that already exists. Astrology allows us to see our surroundings and not gaslight ourselves into seeing something that is not there.

When we look at healing through the lens of astrology, it helps to think about it like a car's make and model, the road we are traveling on, the map we are using, the destination we are traveling to, and the roadblocks we'll encounter. In this chapter, I will guide you to see your chart as a map for understanding and healing through your story. This also helps you begin to prepare for the magic that is yet to come once you unlock these placements in your chart.

Before we move forward, let's talk a bit about the whole sign versus Placidus house systems. I want you to close your eyes and visualize the sky divided into twelve equal parts, known as houses. Now the sky is a 360-degree pie. It's sliced into twelve equal sections, each representing a different area of our lives. Whole sign astrology is one of the earliest house systems, dating to the Hellenistic era, and many people refer to whole sign astrology as Hellenistic astrology. These houses are like stages on which the planets act, influencing many aspects of our human existence, including our identity, personal resources, ancestors, relationships, and careers. Each house is aligned with one of the twelve zodiac signs, starting with Aries and ending with Pisces.

Placidus is a common house system, which is a time-based technique for estimating houses, and everything works by house cusps. I prefer whole sign astrology because it's easier to visualize and gives a more accurate depiction of the current transits and energies within the stars. In addition, I have given and experienced more accurate readings with this system. When looking up your astrological chart, I recommend using the tropical zodiac and whole sign house system. The tropical zodiac is the most commonly used in Western astrology and aligns with the seasons, offering clarity on personal growth and life patterns. Whole sign houses, on the other hand, simplify the chart by assigning one sign to each house, making it easier to interpret overarching themes and placements in your life. This combination provides a clear and accessible framework for understanding your chart.

If you're new to astrology, it can be incredibly enlightening to start by looking up your own birth chart. The many online resources and tools make it easy to generate your chart and provide basic interpretations. This can give you a solid foundation and help you become familiar with your sun, moon, and rising signs, as well as the positions of other key planets. However, if you want a deeper, more personalized understanding, a professional astrologer can be invaluable. An astrologer can offer nuanced insights and connect the dots in ways that might not be immediately obvious. They can help you understand complex aspects and transits, providing guidance tailored to your unique life path. Whether you start on your own or with an astrologer, the journey of exploring your chart is a powerful tool for self-discovery and growth.

Reexamining Your Chart

MOST OF US HAVE BEEN TAUGHT to live by our sun signs and what the sun is doing. As beautiful as the sun can be during your healing process, it can also be hard to see the sun and its beauty. So, looking at my past, present, and future, I've used other astrological elements to help me see clearly through the canyon.

Astrology is a review of the combination of planets, stars, progressions, and transits that are connected to your birth date and time. Astrology has ancient roots and has been adapted by many cultures, dating back to the ancient Greeks and early Chinese. Astrologists have mapped and explained historical events in our society. Many cultures use astrology to determine when and who to marry, when and where to move, and even how to forecast changes within a business. Financier J. P. Morgan was once quoted saying that millionaires don't use astrology, but billionaires do. Former

First Lady Nancy Reagan oversaw her husband's schedule through the lens of astrology. It was known that she wouldn't even let the president fly if it wasn't approved by her astrologers. Nancy was adamant that all major decisions and events would be done in consultation with astrological timing.

So, if astrology is helpful for US presidents, maybe it has the power to help us all. One of the most famous studies about astrology reported on a phenomenon known as the Mars effect. The Mars effect was articulated in the 1950s by Michel Gauquelin. The French statistician examined the birth times of very successful athletes and concluded that Mars was in one of two key positions in each athlete's chart. It was either the rising sign or the midheaven. Many criticized the study because they didn't know if the birth times were accurate. Though there were inconsistences, Gauquelin had managed to replicate his results repeatedly. At one point, other scientists hid the results because they didn't want the world to think that Gauquelin was right, but even now you can look at the charts of many successful athletes and see the correlation to Mars in their charts.

The stars truly offer us an exploration of our inner world, charting our life's challenges and joys but also our purpose—showing us who we are amid the vastness of the universe. One of the ways I use astrology is to connect the dots between the events of my life and the forces guiding them, showing me how my life has ebbed and flowed and offering me the wisdom behind my life's path. There are certain indicators that pinpoint when certain things might happen or have happened, offering us the "why" behind the event.

Now let's look at how astrology can help you heal the past, embrace the present, and prepare for your future through a healed lens.

The Four Placements of Healing

WHEN I STARTED LEARNING ABOUT ASTROLOGY, I realized that the celestial bodies that were most integral to understanding our traumas and guiding us on our healing journey were not the ones we usually think about: Chiron (the asteroid), the moon, Jupiter, and your rising sign (ascendant).

As you look at your chart, circle where the following descriptions relate to you and consider how they might now guide you through your healing journey.

Chiron—The Alchemist of the Soul

When we travel through the canyon, we must address our past before we can look forward. To surrender to the map of our energies, it's important for us to know what pain we bring into this lifetime. When we travel through the canyon, we get an opportunity to address our past, and Chiron shines a light on those wounds.

Chiron is known as the wounded healer and is named after a centaur in Greek mythology. There are various stories about Chiron, but the most important was that he had all the power to help others but could not heal himself. He tried desperately to heal himself by isolating in a cave, spending years trying to heal—but with no success. He couldn't break past the barriers of his mind or his physical wounds. I imagine that Chiron had the same problem that most of us face when we start down the canyon and begin our healing journey. We can see what needs to be healed because, for many of us, our trauma is generational. It didn't start with us; we are experiencing the repercussions of our lineage. Chiron shines a light on the root of our wounds, and it takes courage and vulnerability to face those wounds. It allows us to see the past through a new lens. We have carried Chiron's wounds within us, and they will still be a source of contention until we heal those parts of ourselves. That's why Chiron holds the keys to unlocking our greatest insecurities and our biggest strengths. Chiron has the power to show us how we were hurt in the past and how we can heal in this lifetime.

Chiron connects to your personal story of who you are. The Chiron placement and sign in your astrological chart show the origins of the wounds you will heal in this lifetime. The initial wound comes from the origin story of your birth, which we explored in chapter 1. This wound is where you might feel the most inadequate. Chiron motivates you to answer the question of surrendering and allowing ease, showing you where your trauma stems from and the patterns you will constantly deal with until you heal that part of yourself.

Chiron

Take a look at how each Chiron placement can motivate you to keep going through the canyon.

- For the cardinal Chiron signs (Aries, Cancer, Libra, and Capricorn), the wounds they are healing through the canyon are those around the relationships they have with themselves and others. Those relationship wounds concern self-identity, family, home, and partnerships (platonic, romantic, and professional). When they enter the canyon, they will feel a need to mend these relationships to move forward in their personal healing. The emotions run deep with cardinal Chiron signs, and their intense feelings can at times overtake them, making it harder for them to see the forest from the trees. Their journey through the canyon gives them greater self-awareness and self-realization toward the wounds they need to heal. For those with the cardinal Chiron in Aries, the path they tread through life's metaphorical canyon is deeply personal and intricately tied to the realm of relationships—with themselves and with the world around them. As they navigate this canyon, they have a profound urge to reconcile and heal relationships, which is crucial for their personal evolution and healing. Cardinal Chiron souls experience emotions with profound depth, and at times their intense feelings can momentarily cloud their vision, making it challenging to perceive the bigger picture—like struggling to see the forest for the trees. Yet it is this very journey through the canyon that fosters greater self-awareness and realization, guiding them toward recognizing and healing the deep-seated wounds that lie within. This path, though arduous, is a beautiful process of becoming, filled with lessons of self-discovery and the healing power of introspection.

- For the fixed Chiron signs (Taurus, Leo, Scorpio, and Aquarius), the wounds they are healing through the canyon are those connected to generational and inherited trauma. Fixed Chiron signs will also deal with self-worth issues, depending on the archetypes of the communities they were raised in or born into. These wounds are not just surface scratches; they are profound, embedded in the very fabric of their being, and often demand a journey into the somatic depths of their subconscious to unearth and confront. If left unaddressed, the pain from these deep-seated wounds can manifest physically, becoming symptoms of the soul's unrest. The task at hand for these resilient souls is to discover and embrace methods to release this trapped emotional energy, to allow it to flow freely from their bodies, liberating themselves from the weight of the past. This path, while challenging, is a transformative process that calls for introspection, courage, and the willingness to heal not just the self, but the lineage they carry.

- The mutable Chiron signs (Gemini, Virgo, Sagittarius, and Pisces) are healing wounds of truth and authenticity through the canyon. Blessed with the gift of adaptability, mutable Chiron signs can effortlessly resonate with the energies and needs of those around them, yet they often encounter challenges when trying to align with their own energies and core truths. Within the canyon, their path becomes a deeply personal pilgrimage, an opportunity to dive into the depths of their being, to nurture and heal their own wounds with tender care. This journey is driven by a deep-seated desire to understand the essence of their life and the mysteries that life itself holds. However, this quest for growth and self-discovery can sometimes lead them to feel isolated or misunderstood, especially if they find themselves surrounded by individuals who may not share their commitment to personal evolution and understanding. Despite these challenges, their journey is one of immense personal growth, leading them toward a more authentic and truthful existence.

Chiron highlights the areas in your life that will lead to the most challenging parts of the canyon for you, but it also shows you how your pain can be transformative, making you more resilient. Once you work through your own wounds, you gain wisdom and are able to help others with similar struggles. Your wounds have a spiritual component, and healing them allows you to learn the lessons and make peace with your flaws and vulnerabilities, integrating these parts into your healing experience. Your Chiron allows you to bridge between the physical world and source.

Here are some questions to consider as you relate to your Chiron placement:

1. Imagine your intuition is a compass guiding you through life. Perhaps lately, the needle seems stuck. What areas of your life (relationships, self-doubt, finding your purpose) might be linked to your Chiron placement and causing this glitch?
2. Think of a dream, feeling, or thought that keeps popping up. How might this be connected to your Chiron wound? Could it be a key to unlocking deeper healing?
3. Every wound holds a hidden strength. What surprising talent or resilience might be buried beneath your Chiron pain?
4. Have you noticed a pattern in your life that holds you back? How might this be connected to your Chiron wound, and what small step can you take to break free from this cycle?
5. Sometimes, the loudest voice in your head isn't the most helpful. What soothing message or mantra can you repeat to yourself when facing the challenges of your Chiron wound?

Moon—The Emotional Landscape

Oh, the moon. The moon is your emotional landscape through the canyon. Understanding your moon sign helps you become more aware of your emotional needs and patterns while you are healing. It is linked to your past, your childhood experiences, and how you cope emotionally in your relationships—romantic, platonic, and familial. Your connection to your moon is crucial to healing your wounds and navigating the canyon. The moon focuses on the present because when it comes to surrender and acceptance in this lifetime, your emotions might rule you, but they can also give you the skills to heal your current situation.

Your moon sign helps you nourish what your soul needs currently and provides the proper self-care to claim your emotional identity in this lifetime. It is the gateway to how you can turn your dreams into reality. It's how you communicate in your relationships, how you feel safe and seen, and how you gain a sense of accomplishment. I believe that your moon sign also guides your values. It sets the tone for the spiritual and emotional gains in your life. Your moon sign is your subconscious wants, needs, and desires. It is what you consider home and how you nurture yourself and others. Your moon sign is your internal compass, which guides you in the outside world, motivating change and communicating to your soul when it's on the right path and when it's not.

In comparison to your sun sign, which describes how you behave, the moon is what someone sees when they connect with you on an emotional level. Because the moon changes zodiac signs every two or two and a half days, passing through all twelve signs of the zodiac every twenty-seven days or so, it gives you your most present emotional energy and how you feel on a daily basis. Your moon sign is the engine that fuels your emotions and helps you navigate how people respond to you, offering access to the most intimate parts of you and your hidden motivations. When you are thinking about your moon sign as a means to your present, the moon allows you to rectify the past and know what to bring forward with you into the future. When you focus on your moon sign, you tap into a powerful tool for understanding your present situation. The moon encourages you to look back at your past not with regret but with the intention of healing and growing. It presents you with all of your experiences and says this is what serves you and this is what holds you back.

The moon monitors your emotions and offers healing, growth, and transformation, and it shows you how to be present in your day-to-day moments. Let's see how each moon modality deals with the canyon on a present level.

Moon

- For the cardinal moon signs (Aries, Cancer, Libra, and Capricorn), navigating through the canyon is like embarking on a journey of continual rebirths where each step forward is seen as an opportunity to start anew. They find a certain thrill in the concept of beginning again, embracing change with open arms. The cardinal moon signs naturally set the emotional climate for themselves and for those in their orbit, crafting an environment that not only nurtures but also instills a sense of discipline and structure, making their passage through the canyon smoother and more harmonious than most. Their intuitive grasp of the emotional landscape around them offers a distinct edge, allowing them to navigate their spiritual quests, relationships, and professional endeavors with a keen insight and understanding. This heightened sensitivity to their emotional environment empowers them to lead, inspire, and achieve their aspirations with grace and resilience.
- When the fixed moon signs (Taurus, Leo, Scorpio, and Aquarius) travel through the canyon, they view their emotional well-being as a predictable emotional rhythm. Their approach to emotional well-being is about finding a method that resonates deeply with them, and once it has been discovered, they dedicate themselves

to nurturing routines and habits that safeguard their emotional equilibrium. The fixed moon signs are architects of their own emotional sanctuaries, establishing firm boundaries that act not only as shields but also as the foundation upon which they can securely explore and expand their emotional depths. However, their natural resilience and commitment to stability can sometimes manifest as resistance to change, holding steadfast until the weight of remaining the same surpasses the discomfort of transformation. It is within these moments of inevitable shift that their true strength emerges. Confronted by discomfort, they are propelled into a period of introspection and renewal, seizing control of their emotional journey. This process of reflection and adaptation becomes a powerful catalyst for profound personal growth and transformation, marking a pivotal point in their emotional evolution.

- For the mutable moon signs (Gemini, Virgo, Sagittarius, and Pisces), the passage through the canyon is a deeply spiritual act of communication, one that transcends mere words and allows them to connect and express their emotions with profound clarity. This unique ability to articulate their innermost feelings facilitates deeper connections with those they encounter, enhancing the effectiveness of their healing journey. The mutable moon signs possess an innate problem-solving prowess coupled with a remarkable resilience and an openness to change. This flexibility is their superpower, enabling them to navigate new paths and recover from emotional challenges with grace. Their journey is one of constant evolution, where setbacks are not roadblocks but rather stepping stones to greater understanding and personal growth. Through this adaptive and communicative approach, they are able to weave a rich tapestry of emotional well-being that is both healing and transformative.

Astrology

As you journey through this part of the canyon, your moon becomes your inner security and builds an inner stability that is vital for you as you address deeper emotional wounds. Allow your moon to offer you insight into your subconscious patterns and behaviors and any underlying issues that affect you negatively. Allow your moon to help you foster a deeper connection to your soul.

Here are a few questions to ponder as you're considering your moon:

1. Within the canyon walls, sound bounces endlessly. How do you think your emotions might echo there? Do strong feelings get easily amplified, or do you struggle to pick up on subtle emotional cues? How can you be more mindful of these echoes during your healing journey?
2. Forget north. Imagine a compass guiding you toward emotional well-being within the canyon. What internal signal or intuition guides you when navigating your emotions? How can you learn to trust and follow this inner compass?
3. A wide emotional chasm appears within the canyon. How would you bridge this gap to connect with the other side? Would you rely on clear communication, shared experiences, or empathy to connect?
4. Sometimes the most valuable messages come as whispers. Recall a time you felt a strong emotional pull but couldn't understand it. How might you become more receptive to these subtle emotional cues within the canyon?
5. Within the canyon, you encounter a well-worn path and an overgrown path through dense, unexplored forest. Which path feels more comfortable? Do you find comfort in familiar routines, or are

you energized by exploring new emotional territory? How can you leverage this strength during your journey?

Jupiter—The Blessing

Jupiter—the planet of fortune, expansion, blessings, and favor—is how we heal the future and surrender to it with ease. In some circles, Jupiter is known as Santa Claus or the Great Benefic. It shows us where we have the greatest opportunity for growth and how we can focus during Jupiter transits. Jupiter can also provide us with the spiritual wisdom and freedom needed to influence our lives. Jupiter gives us the faith to look toward our future and shows which direction we should go to gain the most spiritually. It has the power to pique our curiosity and get the answers to many of life's questions.

When I first discovered my Jupiter sign, which is in Libra, it explained many of my interests and dreams. At the beginning of my healing journey, I never paid attention to how big a role my natal and transiting house of Jupiter played in the themes I was experiencing.

But Jupiter has been a game changer in how I expand and surrender to what is and what can be. Jupiter gives you the tools to see outside of yourself, whereas your moon and Chiron tap into your emotional journey within. Jupiter says, *I want you to flourish and live your best life and stay on the path where you can feel the most seen and heard.* Jupiter allows you to have an optimistic view about your life, which is crucial to overcoming challenges, encouraging you to broaden your horizons and look at the bigger picture.

Having this expanded perspective helps you understand and heal from your experiences.

Jupiter

- For the cardinal Jupiter signs (Aries, Cancer, Libra, and Capricorn), when it comes to their outlook on their healing journey through the canyon, they can adapt and are able to handle emotional wounds while seeking solutions to help them thrive when under emotional pressure. These souls are not just survivors; they are seekers of solutions, constantly exploring ways to transform their lifestyle and mindset to not only cope with but flourish under emotional duress. Their pursuit is not merely about healing; it's about thriving amidst the challenges. This optimistic outlook is at the core of their being, fueling a belief in the promise of better days ahead. As they traverse the more daunting segments of the canyon, their resilience becomes a beacon of hope and inspiration for those around them. Cardinal signs possess a unique blend of courage and foresight, enabling them to see beyond the immediate struggle, envisioning a future where their current trials have shaped them into stronger, more compassionate beings. This visionary perspective is a testament to their ability to lead by example, demonstrating the power of resilience and optimism in the face of life's inevitable ebbs and flows.
- For those with fixed Jupiter signs (Taurus, Leo, Scorpio, and Aquarius), the path through the canyon is navigated with a therapeutic and introspective lens. This journey is not about quick fixes or surface-level healing; instead, it's a deep dive into the heart of their emotional landscape. Armed with an analytical and reflective mind, these individuals are adept at uncovering the roots of their challenges, favoring a profound understanding over fleeting relief. The wisdom inherent in fixed Jupiter signs is their ability to transform pain into purposeful insight, viewing each experience as

a lesson to be learned and integrated. This process is not just about healing; it's about evolving, turning their trials into treasures of wisdom that guide their way. As they journey through the canyon, their deeply held beliefs and values serve as an anchor, providing stability and direction amid the flux of emotional healing.

- For the mutable Jupiter signs (Gemini, Virgo, Sagittarius, and Pisces), the healing journey through the canyon is characterized by an unparalleled adaptability and flexibility. This journey is fluid, with paths that twist and turn, demanding a versatile approach to emotional healing. These individuals are masters of adjustment, able to refine and evolve their healing practices in harmony with their ever-changing circumstances, showcasing an impressive dexterity in navigating the emotional landscape. Mutable Jupiter signs possess a profound connection to both their spirituality and creativity, making these realms powerful conduits for emotional release and catharsis. Their depth of understanding and intuition allows them to engage with their emotions on a deeply intuitive level, facilitating a healing process that is both transformative and deeply aligned with their true essence.

Your Jupiter sign represents your spiritual exploration and search for meaning in this lifetime. Jupiter's energy helps you let go of grudges and move toward forgiveness, building your self-belief while you heal through the canyon. Your self-belief is what you will need when your journey gets tough and when you are faced with insecurities. Once you learn how to track your Jupiter sign, you can attract opportunities for growth and healing that may not have been open to you in the past.

Here are some questions to consider in relationship to your Jupiter:

1. A steep mountain rises within the canyon. How would you approach this challenge? Do you see it as an obstacle to overcome with a head-on charge or as an opportunity for growth through ascent to a higher perspective?
2. You encounter a cryptic inscription on a canyon wall. Would you rely solely on your own analysis to understand its meaning or seek guidance from others for external solutions? How can you leverage both approaches during your healing journey?
3. A cleansing waterfall cascades within the canyon. How would you utilize this natural resource to release emotional burdens? Do you find creative expression (like artistic catharsis) or spiritual practices (like soul cleansing) to be more effective for emotional release?
4. You encounter a symbolic representation of a past hurt within the canyon. How would you approach this encounter? Would you focus on extracting valuable lessons from the experience, learning from the past, or prioritize letting go of resentment and granting forgiveness?
5. A resilient wildflower blooms within a rocky crevice of the canyon. How does this image resonate with your healing journey? Do you see yourself developing unwavering resilience to navigate challenges, building inner strength, and actively transforming your emotional landscape to blossom into a new version of yourself?

Your Rising Sign—The Soul's Shield

Your rising sign, also known as the ascendant, was ascending on the eastern horizon at the time of your birth. It plays a significant role while you are doing your canyon work because it shapes your personality, your appearance, and how you show up in the world—or as I like to say, it's the human vessel our soul chose for walking through this lifetime, and it's our outer warrior that protects us. It's the lens through which we see the canyon, determining how we will face our fears and heal ourselves. It will guide how we react to the canyon's environment.

Your ascendant gives you insights about how you cope and work through patterns, both healthy and unhealthy ones. It also influences how you are perceived by others. It is the shield that protects your ego self, which can be seen as your sun sign. Your rising sign also dictates your emotional resilience, which is key for doing your work through the canyon; resilience prepares you for the obstacles and how you navigate your life's purpose. The various rising signs offer us guidance on how we move through the canyon and through this world.

Rising/Ascendant

- For the fixed rising signs (Taurus, Leo, Scorpio, and Aquarius), the passage through the canyon is characterized by a steadfast focus and a quiet determination. They have a rhythm, a kind of soulful consistency that guides their journey; it's their healing dance, and they commit to it with a deep sense of loyalty. Their dedication to their healing process isn't just a part of the journey, it's the very thing that will make the path clearer and their strides more assured. They don't just participate in their journey—they infuse it with a raw authenticity and a profound commitment that is uniquely theirs. And when they face obstacles, as long as they don't let that innate stubborn streak obscure the way, fixed rising signs have the capacity to tap into a well of emotional depth that is rare and transformative. Their journey through the canyon isn't just about reaching the other side; it's about discovering the vastness within themselves, a depth that is as formidable as it is beautiful.

- For the cardinal rising signs (Aries, Cancer, Libra, and Capricorn), when it comes to traveling through the canyon, they can adapt and venture into new horizons. They are natural initiators. Their journey through the canyon is one of courageous initiation and exploration into new realms of being. These souls don't just traverse paths; they forge them with a pioneering spirit that breathes life into their every step. Their approach to healing and growth weaves a complex tapestry that intertwines the many facets of their existence, embracing a holistic perspective that honors the union of mind, body, and spirit. Cardinal rising signs have an affinity for the path less traveled—alternative therapies, the ancient wisdom of yoga, and any practice that breaks away from conventional paradigms. Their healing process is not a solitary trek but a collective voyage that is enriched by the shared wisdom and support of a community.
- For the mutable rising signs (Gemini, Virgo, Sagittarius, and Pisces), the voyage through the canyon is graced with a natural agility and an innate capacity for deep emotional understanding. This blend of adaptability and emotional intelligence, coupled with an insatiable curiosity for the spiritual dimensions of life, equips them with a unique set of tools for healing and self-improvement. When mutable rising signs fully commit to their personal odyssey, they unlock an extraordinary dynamic within their healing journey. It's their inherent flexibility and willingness to entertain diverse philosophies that not only allow them to thrive but also to navigate the healing process with an ease that seems almost like a dance—an ever-changing, ever-flowing movement toward wholeness. Their path is a testament to the power of openness, learning, and transformation.

The rising sign is critical to your soul's journey through the canyon, offering you the lens through which you look at life, especially in the toughest times. Your rising sign is your soul's vibration. It guides your energy, helping you maintain balance and avoid healing burnout. Your ascendant is also the gateway to your spiritual awakening, offering new pathways for growth.

Here are some questions to consider while you're exploring your rising sign:

1. A hidden path branches off from the main trail within the canyon. How comfortable are you venturing off the beaten track? Does your rising sign crave stability and routine, sticking to the familiar trail, or do you find excitement in exploring uncharted territory, taking the hidden path?
2. A crystal-clear pool reflects your image within the canyon. How comfortable are you with what you see? Does your rising sign make you prioritize presenting a confident persona, a polished reflection, or are you open to exploring your vulnerabilities and embracing your true reflection?
3. Boulders block your path within the canyon. How would you approach this challenge? Does your rising sign make you persistent and determined, removing the boulders, or do you seek creative solutions to navigate around them, finding a new way forward?
4. You encounter different food sources within the canyon—some familiar and comforting, others exotic and unknown. How would you choose what to nourish yourself with? Does your rising sign make you crave stability and comfortable, familiar foods, or are you open to trying new things to fuel your journey, exploring the unknown?
5. You encounter a rare and beautiful flower within the canyon. How does it embody the essence of your healing journey? Does

your rising sign highlight your unwavering strength, like a resilient flower, or your capacity for growth and transformation, like a blooming flower?

Embodying Your Astrology

HAVE YOU HEARD OF THE 80/20 RULE? It's also known as the Pareto principle: that 80 percent of our outcomes come from 20 percent of our inputs. Well, similarly, I believe that all these modalities—astrology, human design, numerology, etc.—are 80 percent accurate, and the remaining 20 percent of life's outcomes are influenced by how we were raised, our socioeconomic status, the traumas we endured, and our personal origin stories. We can get stuck looking at our lives just from that 20 percent lens and live from there for as long as we choose to.

Even though the man who raised me worked for himself and was extremely successful at multiple ventures, I was pushed toward business and to get a job, rather than pursue the creative aspirations I had had since I was a child. When I was growing up, I dreamed of going to LA and attending film school because I wanted to be a screenwriter and film producer, but my parents didn't think that was a viable career. Instead, my parents' influence led me to choose business school. My guides, my stars, and my inner channeling told me a different story—the 80 percent of my life's destiny—but I chose to listen to the 20 percent and found myself in a deep misalignment.

As I began to dive deeper into my natal chart and the placements, I realized that I had the power to change my perspective and to not let my conditioning get in the way of my true calling and destiny.

Astrology is a gift and the blueprint for how you move in the world, offering you guidance to create ease and abundance, but most importantly, it allows you to heal and understand why you've been sent in the direction you are choosing. There is a saying that what you want wants you, and I truly believe that spirit never puts any goal or dream in your heart that you are not meant to have. The trick is to get out of the way and allow it and lean in to the essence of your true self and your calling.

Some of us don't answer the call when it's presented to us in our life, and we keep going and pushing past what we truly want and desire. But when we ignore our soul's calling, we find ourselves out of alignment and out of joy.

We have chosen the path that we are on, but the issue many of us face, including myself, is whether we are going to listen to the guidance we receive along the way. My last few years in corporate America were pure hell. In the early stages of my career, I loved sales because I was good at it. I knew how to build relationships with people to get them to buy into me. But then I went through a series of job losses, and it started feeling overwhelming. It was like I couldn't keep a job, and time after time, I knew deep in my heart that it was because this wasn't what I was supposed to do—or who I was supposed to be.

I knew I had a calling in my life to be a spiritual teacher and to use my psychic gifts to help others. I remember being asked to lunch by coworkers so I could give them readings. It was flattering, but I needed to pay my bills, so I remained in dead-end jobs to "support" myself, but they always ended. Finally, in my last corporate job, I had to look at myself in the mirror and say, *You must bet on yourself.* And once I did, I never looked back.

But this was always written in the stars. Every astrologer would tell me, "You need to work for yourself" and "You're going to work for yourself one day." But I couldn't see it. Finally, I decided to embrace everything in my chart and lean in to what I've known all along. It hasn't been easy, but it's been right.

Astrology may not lead you to entrepreneurship, but the path is written in the stars and offers you a healing path toward yourself. Imagine being a spirit and choosing what time you would come into the world because the stars would align at certain times for you to fulfill your destiny and purpose. Through astrology, we have the ability to see that life story through a different lens.

When we can embody self, we are able to fulfill our destinies or at least be open to what our destinies might bring. It gives us the space to be ourselves and embrace the parts that we may have been taught or been conditioned to ignore or leave behind due to religion, socioeconomic status, or education.

Embodying self requires us to show up fully and unapologetically as ourselves, but that can be hard when we are taught to conform to certain ways of being. When you embody self, you learn to embrace your values and stand firm in who you are without any outside influences. And astrology can guide you to surrender to those deep and powerful truths.

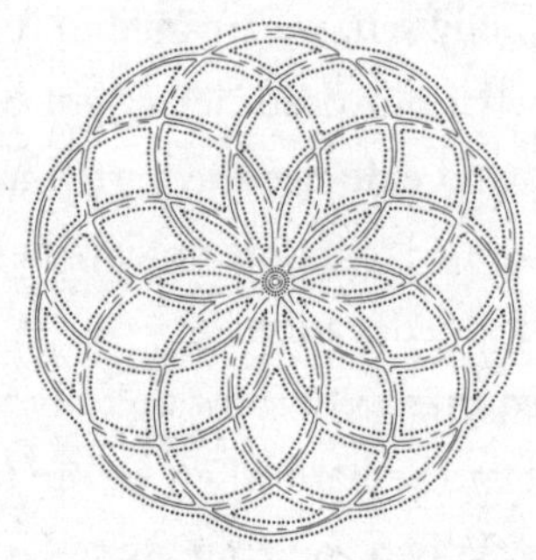

What's Not Aligning in My Life, Business, or Career?

4

NUMEROLOGY

The Embodiment of Alignment

AISHA, GRAB ME A PEN off the counter," my grandma would yell across the kitchen at me while she sat next to the phone and read off her numbers to the man from the number spot. "302, 225, 103, 179, 484, 1020," and so on. I would give her a pen, and she would write on a piece of paper all the numbers that she said, and then I would look at her and say, "Don't forget 310," which is my birthday. That would trigger her to play a few other birthdays in the family. "Let me have 811, 314, and 428 boxed for fifty cents." Then she'd be on to the pick-four numbers, and she would hang up the phone and prepare for the day. Depending on the numbers she played, we would go either that day or the day after to pick up her money. Either way, she would hit.

I don't remember my life without numbers. From my grandmother's gambling to numbers symbolizing energy, numbers have been part of the inner makings of me. My grandmother's phone was like a hotline for birthdays and times of birth. Anytime a baby was born in the family, someone would call my grandmother just to tell her the birth date and time so she could put it in her Bible. I would hear her say, "That's a good number" or "A good day to be born on." Numbers in my family were so important that I remember my father selecting the numbers for new phone lines. I would hear him talking to the phone company: "You don't have another number, maybe something that ends in an eight or a five?" This was protocol.

My family knew numbers had energy behind them. Numbers are special. It's no coincidence that my cousin and I were born on the same day years apart. It's no coincidence that where you live holds an energy related to how you feel. It's no coincidence that the day you were born dictates the energies that are within you and unfold over time as you become more self-actualized.

Numerology is all around us. The numbers matter. These numbers are what keep you in alignment with those natural energies of your soul. I make sure that I use numerology in many of the things that I do. It's more than a ritual for me. It's how I was taught. It's part of my ancestral lineage. The energy of numerology can be a catalyst not only for growth but for healing. Every number is connected to something.

Whether it's a planet, a zodiac, the divine masculine or feminine, or an element, it's all connected. Numerology is a fascinating way to gain insights into your life by understanding the vibrational significance of numbers. To start, you can explore the core numbers in your numerology chart, such as your life path number.

For example, to find your life path number, add the digits of your birth date together until you get a single digit. If you were born on July 19, 1985, for example, you would calculate it like this: 7 (July) + 1 + 9 (day) + 1 + 9 + 8 + 5 (year) = 40. Then, add 4 + 0 to get 4. So, your life path number would be 4.

After a long-term relationship ended, I moved into an apartment, the number of which added up to the number 1. I had never lived in a number 1 home, and I didn't expect and wasn't prepared for what came with living there. Living in a number 1 home gave me the opportunity to step into my independence as a true adult. Since I had just left a five-year relationship and had been living with my ex, I had freedom to be who I truly was.

My ex and I grew up in very different environments, and we had very different values. How that played out led to us growing apart even though I don't think we were ever truly on the same page. Society put pressure on our relationship to be on pace with what our peers were doing, when all along we really didn't have the same vision for our lives.

Living in this place was new and exciting, and I was motivated to prove my ex wrong and show myself that I could make it on my own. This number 1 home even gave me the courage to lean in to my creativity, showcasing my talents through entrepreneurship. At the time, I had a successful product-based business that was getting press in national magazines and earning celebrity endorsements, but it also turned my home into a factory. I was overworked and stressed. I didn't truly know what balance was until I moved. The new apartment felt like I was attracting lots of abundance when that wasn't always the case. Yes, I've had a lot of high moments there, but I've also had some very low lows. I never quite understood how to balance the energies of living in a number 1 home. I learned how to foster community, but I didn't know how to create a relaxing environment.

I felt like I was spending more time surviving, trying to make it on my own, than thriving in community and abundance, I felt myself leaning in to a very unhealthy masculine energy, and I didn't like it.

I knew that this energy was overtaking me, and I had to get out of it and move. But I found myself entering into another canyon. I was changing, moving out of the space of the hyper-independence and loneliness that are a huge part of being an only child. But change can be hard. I felt unaligned like I never had before.

While you are in the canyon, you'll understand how numerology can keep you on the path that your soul has come to experience. At times we think that we are just moving in a direction of our free will. But as an old-school spiritual teacher named Joan Pancoe once said, free will is god/spirit telling you to stand on one foot and allowing you to choose which foot to stand on. When you are out of alignment with your numerological energies, you feel it. You feel it in your daily life, in your relationships, and in your career. When you continue to go against the grain of your natural energetic being, you feel like a fish out of water praying that someone comes along and throws you back into the ocean where you feel at home. When you ignore the numerical essence of who you are, you will always be trying to find your way back home. This feeling lingers with you until you decide to align with your numbers.

Walking in Alignment with Your Path

ALIGNMENT IS BEING IN HARMONY WITH the true nature of your soul's spirit. Alignment allows you to self-actualize into your purpose. By aligning your thoughts, actions, and beliefs with your values and goals, you will experience clarity and fulfillment within your life. Being in alignment allows you to be one with nature and the universal laws. If I were to ask you, "What brings you inner peace and happiness?" would you know the answer?

It was a cold winter night on November 8, 2016, and I was in a "situationship." I was still living with my ex because we had signed a new lease, and I was just beginning to look for a new place. In the meantime, we had started living two separate lives in our two-bedroom home. On the eve of the 2016 election, as the votes were coming in from each state, I and my situationship decided to take a pause from the election. It looked as though our world was going to be in shambles in the morning—a reality TV star was about to be elected president.

We had passionate unprotected soul-tie sex just as the news was coming in about the new president.

It didn't take long for me to find out I was pregnant because my body felt different the morning after. An energy that I had never felt before was emanating from my womb. My cycle was due to start in a few days, but it never came. Eight days later, I took a pregnancy test, and it was positive.

I'd never been pregnant before. I wasn't necessarily scared, but I knew my situationship was unreliable and new—and I was technically still living with my ex-boyfriend. Like many things in my life at that time, I didn't know what I was going to do. I never thought I could conceive because I had been diagnosed with polycystic ovary syndrome, or PCOS, a hormonal disorder common among women of reproductive age. PCOS is characterized by irregular menstrual periods, excess androgen levels, and polycystic ovaries that can lead to various health challenges. I was shocked about the pregnancy, but more shocked that I conceived on that election night. For a few weeks I enjoyed being pregnant—the estrogen and progesterone levels made me feel euphoric—but reality set in quickly. I made the decision to have an abortion. The only place I felt safe going to was Planned Parenthood. So, I called and made an appointment. I went there and we scheduled the day for the procedure.

For the next week and a half, I was having the most up and down emotions. I was starting to regret making the appointment. I moved into my new apartment two days before my scheduled abortion, but something interesting happened. I started bleeding. Not a heavy bleeding but just spotting. The bleeding stopped and I headed to Planned Parenthood by myself. My blood pressure was sky high, and when the nurse called me in to get a sonogram, she didn't see anything. She asked whether I had been bleeding anytime before that day. I said yes. She confirmed I was having a miscarriage; I was relieved.

This is why the personal years in numerology are so important. For some reason, I felt like god knew I wouldn't be able to deal with myself if I had gone through with it. And in numerology, that is what we refer to as a personal year 4. Your personal year number offers insight into the themes and experiences you might encounter throughout the year. To calculate it, simply add your birth month and day to the current year. For example, if your birthday is March 1 and the current year is 2025, you would add 3 (March) + 1 (day) + 2 + 0 + 2 + 5 (year) = 13. Then, add 1 + 3 to get 4. So, 2025 would be a personal year 4 for you. This number can help guide your actions and decisions, aligning you with the natural flow of the year's energy.

A personal year 4 in numerology is what I call the "if your shit is not together, the universe will force you to get it together" year. The personal year 4 is all about building a strong foundation. It asks you to find out where things are unstable in your life and where you need to be more disciplined. It creates a foundation for success, and if you aren't willing to prioritize your well-being, you will have a hard time thriving in all areas.

One of the interesting things that can happen during a personal year 4 is that your free will gets tested, and you can feel boxed in by circumstances that are beyond your control. Part of me was sad. I had dodged getting pregnant with exes before when we had "slip-ups," and I didn't know if I would ever get pregnant again because it had not happened before. I had to face the fact that a personal year 4 can get hard, and the only way forward is through—this is how I've been able to accept alignment in my life: knowing that spirit is in control even in the moments when I am confused and not sure of the direction I need to go.

Spirit's alignment, made clear through numerology, always leads the way. For those new to numerology, it's important to understand that this practice reveals the underlying patterns and energies in your life. By calculating and interpreting key numbers like your life path and personal year, you can gain profound insights and direction. Your life path number gives you an overview of your life's purpose and core strengths, while your personal year number highlights the themes and opportunities specific to the current year, making it easier to navigate life's challenges and opportunities.

Alignment with spirit allows you to surrender to what is and operate at your highest capacity within that alignment, understanding the energy, season, and weather of your own life. Without this knowledge, we could step out into winter wearing a swimsuit or walk out into the rain without an umbrella.

This has happened to me many times, especially in relationships with the wrong people, but those relationships led me to ask better questions and get clearer about myself and my boundaries. I had to learn from these relationships that my needs mattered. In a strange way, that was foreign to me. As a child, walking on eggshells so I wouldn't get yelled at was a way of life for me. I had to learn that it's perfectly fine to get my needs met and that if people cannot meet my needs, then it's also okay to walk away.

Everything wrong will lead you to everything right. All roads lead to alignment. That's why there is no wrong way; there is only a way. At the time, it might feel as though you have ruined your life or that you will never find another love or friend or job, but all roads lead you to the right people—the right jobs and career, the right friendships, and the right relationships, even the right situationships. Nothing is done in vain. Nothing is by mistake. With that awareness, will you accept that what you feel and grow through is going to get you to your promised land, or will you continue to fight against the nature of all things? Will you continue to force things and try to fit together things that don't belong together? Can you accept that you can grow through anything, purposefully and in alignment with your life's path? And yes, this applies to the hardest things too, the greatest losses and pains and grief.

Instead of trying to control what happens, focus on the person you want to be while you are growing through the thing. Focus on the lessons you want to learn about yourself. Set intentions to hold space for the new versions of yourself at every opportunity you get. And that doesn't mean that we don't also take the time to grieve and fall apart and have our times where everything can feel meaningless—but know, that is part of the path too.

With awareness, the alignment will unfold as you live.

By creating intentions that help you unfold into someone who not only takes life head-on but embraces life with an open heart, you will begin to trust in your own alignment. Give yourself permission to not know what you want. It's okay to be uncertain and to take your time exploring different paths and possibilities, to seek things that feel good today but will not in a month or two. It will all lead you to alignment. It will all lead you to the destination called purpose. You will never know what is supposed to be if you don't feel what you don't want at all. You think you know, but you have no clue. Who you are today will not be the person you will be next year or even next month. As your soul searches for existence and truth, you will constantly evolve. You will constantly uncover more and more truth about yourself.

Alignment is truth. Alignment is not fear and control.

Alignment is freedom—freedom in knowing that your mistakes, mishaps, bad decisions, and impulses will all bring you back to center eventually. When you accept that, you can live a full life, a passionate life, and a life that you will want to tell everyone about.

The alignment many seek now is about controlling the outcome. How can you be the best or jump on the fast track to a destination you don't even know you want in the first place? Stop holding on to false narratives. Embrace the unknown. The magic of alignment makes room for everything your soul is seeking. You must not rush this process; you have to allow it to happen and consume you. Let go of control and let freedom consume you.

The Alignment Compass: The Uncharted Path

THROUGH THE TRIALS AND TRIBULATIONS OF your soul's awakening, you will discover that alignment has always been there. You were always on track to reach your goals and have a clear understanding of who you are journeying to be. When you let go of control, you get an opportunity to invite any possibility that the universe has in mind to make sure you get in alignment with your soul and the desires of your heart, and you begin to build your alignment compass. This exercise will help you shed control, embrace the unknown, and begin aligning yourself with your truest desires.

Alignment Exercise

1. Jot down three things you currently desire. Be honest—these can be anything! Now, circle the one that feels most fleeting, something that might lose its appeal quickly.
2. Why do you want the circled desire? Is it truly fulfilling a deeper need, or is it based on external pressure or temporary pleasure? Write a short paragraph exploring this.
3. Imagine waking up tomorrow completely open-minded. You have no predetermined desires, just a willingness to explore possibilities. How does this feel? Write down any anxieties or feelings of liberation that arise.
4. Draw a large circle on a piece of paper. Inside, write down everything that feels safe and familiar (habits, routines, people). Outside the circle, list things that feel unknown or scary (new experiences, career changes).
5. Close your eyes and imagine venturing outside your comfort zone. What sounds do you hear (city streets, nature sounds)? What sights greet you? Describe the sensations you feel: Are you exhilarated, overwhelmed, or filled with anticipation?
6. Think about your experiences with desires and venturing outside your comfort zone. Did any anxieties or fears surface? What feelings of excitement or possibility emerge? Create a short "soundtrack" that captures the essence of these experiences using music, nature sounds, or affirmations.

Alignment is contentment, as your actions and thoughts are congruent with your personal values and beliefs. You walk with a knowing that no matter what, you have the inner wisdom and intuition to lead you to more confident and concise decision-making. You reach this alignment by addressing and releasing past traumas and emotional wounds, which leads to emotional healing. When we are out of alignment, our bodies can feel the stress and anxiety, and it can physically manifest in health issues. Once you release these negative emotions, you can heal yourself.

Getting It Right

EMBODYING ALIGNMENT THROUGH THE CANYON IS a transformative journey that deeply influences every part of your life. It signals the alignment within your inner world by integrating the parts of yourself that may feel broken or fragmented. When you embrace your journey in the canyon, you confront and process wounds and fears that have embedded burdens within you. Once you acknowledge these wounds, you can reshape your identity and belief system and unleash your most authentic self. In this part of the canyon, it's important for you to acknowledge and integrate the hidden, darker aspects of your soul, which further helps you align. When you bring light to the part of yourself that may have been suppressed and ignored, you are able to become your whole self. You can be in harmonious coexistence with the light and dark parts of yourself.

As you try to find your purpose in life, you will be pulled in different directions, and they will all feel like the right choices. However, you might wake up and notice that you are unfulfilled and joyless about your current position or career. Alignment will make you face your life choices head-on and evaluate everything you've decided up until then. Don't fret. That's the point. That's the mission your soul is on. That is how you can attain the freedom you seek in this lifetime. You are not your career or job, but they most certainly need to be and will be in alignment with who your soul meant you to be in this lifetime.

You might be unhappy with what you are currently doing, but what if that is the way toward alignment?

What if getting aligned only happens after you mess up and make mistakes? What if alignment only comes to pass when you seek the wrong things and make the wrong choices? What if there is no other way? Alignment can only happen if you walk in the wrong direction because it will signal your soul that you are going the wrong way.

For as long as I can remember, I've chased the idea of "getting it right." Because if I didn't, I believed that my environment would blow up. Getting it right was a marker for success (or whatever I had defined as success). But of course, that never felt right. It was as if I were moving my own goalpost time and time again: Graduate with your MBA, find the job that pays you the most, do the things people only dream about.

I knew that it couldn't have been the right way all the time because detours came. Every misstep, every heartbreak, felt like my world was crashing, but all along it was putting me right back into alignment. My perspective changed, and every time I picked myself up from the floor, or uncurled myself from crying in a fetal position, it dawned on me: This discomfort was a signal, not a punishment. It was my soul whispering to me, past all the chaotic mind chatter, *This isn't you or where or what you're supposed to be. Stop forcing things that aren't in alignment for you*. I spent so much time trying to make "fetch" happen for myself that I was missing the flow of what spirit was offering me. But then I began to see the detours as more than lessons. They became my teachers.

My internal compass was recalibrating itself with every single heartache, every single failure. It made me realize that alignment might not come from the perfect path, but rather from the detours that consistently drive us back to the path and redesign it. There is discomfort in nonalignment because it's a powerful opportunity to refine your inner compass as you learn which directions you were meant to go, and when.

As you weave the tapestry of canyon work into your life, you begin to transform in subtle and profound ways. You begin to live with a deeper sense of purpose, and your life begins to reflect the alignment you want, need, and desire. When you are out of alignment, you walk with a cloud that hovers over you, and everything looks as though a storm is brewing even if it's a sunny day filled with birds chirping and crisp air and calm energy. But when you are out of alignment, you have trouble seeing the sun shining and the birds singing. You have trouble seeing anything clearly because you are faced with looking at the world through the lens of pain and trauma. That is not what your soul came to do.

Yes, you will experience unfortunate events, and they will shape you into a person who knows how to let a mean joke roll off your back or allow people to underestimate you. But that is not why you were brought here. Alignment offers you a journey of returning to yourself. By being in alignment with the natural aura of your being, you are here to radiate your soul's purpose and be an example to the lifetimes that will come after you. When you live your life in alignment, you prepare your soul to evolve into something new in the next life.

This experience you are having in this lifetime is not one and done. It's a preparation to evolve into something greater than you could ever imagine. This is where numerology comes in.

Numerology can aid you in helping your soul stay on the right path. Imagine your soul picking an energy that keeps it secure, stable, joyful, and happy, as long you stay in alignment with the energies you were born into. That is how numerology helps you.

The Energy of Numerology

WE CAN USE NUMEROLOGY TO EMBODY alignment in three ways: through our life path number, our personal year number, and the universal year number. I like to say our life path number is the wardrobe we wear in our personal year's weather and in the universal year's season.

We use numerology to embody alignment in a multitude of ways. Numerology is a vibrational understanding between us and the universe. Numbers have a specific frequency, and working with them helps align you to energies that assist in fueling your personal growth and life path. Numerology provides a unique blend of emotional, spiritual, and holistic ways for you to gain a sense of personal awareness as you learn lessons in this lifetime. It serves as a guide offering clarity in times of inaction and indecision. When you embrace the energies at play, you can make choices that support and are in alignment with your most authentic and higher self. When you work with the universal energies instead of against them, you offer your soul a chance to complete its mission and learn the lessons it came here to learn.

When you understand how to work with these energies, you allow yourself to be guided by a mystical presence that leads you to the greatest evolution of self. You become one with universal law. Every number you integrate with holds a frequency, from your address to the letters in your name and even the time you were born. Have you ever noticed that you gravitate toward a certain number or series of numbers? That's not by accident. That is the universe bringing that frequency to your attention to keep you on track. You know what it feels like to go against the grain. It's uncomfortable. Because of trauma and conditioning, we think we must struggle in order to have what we want, need, and desire. But what if you have had the road map all along, and the numbers that you were born into are the pathway to keep you moving in the direction that your soul desires? That path can be easy if you make the decision to just listen and let the frequencies of your soul guide you.

My life path number is 5. I am energetic, adaptable, and love to explore the curiosities of life. New cultures and environments light me up. When I go long periods without traveling or changing my environment, I can feel my body tensing up, and I feel like I'm trapped with nowhere to go. I have learned over the years that to stay in alignment with my true nature I must go and visit a new neighborhood, talk to new people, and experience that world as if I've never been here before so that my soul remains happy in a place of receiving.

Embodying alignment isn't just about staying on this straight and narrow path, it's about putting yourself in a position to receive spirit's abundance for you. To receive means to be given or presented something. It's spirit's way of giving you what you came here to experience. Goodness is your birthright, and using numerology as a tool for goodness can set you free. This doesn't mean that life won't throw you curveballs to kick you out of alignment and throw you off course, but when you feel yourself spiraling, look to the frequencies of your numbers to uplift you and be a guiding light to your humanity.

My French bulldog of ten years died on my birthday approximately one hour after the time I was born. As she was gasping for air while taking her last breaths, I petted her and let her know it was okay to cross over. I thanked her for getting me to my new location—I had just moved to a new state three weeks prior. She looked at me and then closed her eyes, and she was gone. I was hurt and cried my eyes out, but I knew I had given her the best life possible. The numerical symbolism of her crossing over on my birthday was hard at first, but I felt honored at the gift she gave me of transitioning to the rainbow bridge after seeing me settled in my new home.

Her death threw me off, but a few days later, I had the privilege to board a plane to visit Rio de Janeiro for the first time, and I felt as if god knew I needed to get back into alignment. The trip was planned a few weeks in advance, but with my Frenchie being sick, the few weeks before the trip seemed like a blur. For me, birthdays symbolize new beginnings, and her death just three days prior to my departure was a sign that I was on the right path. I was open to receiving the abundance that was offered to me in that moment.

This is why numerology is a powerful tool that allows you to experience spirit in the highest frequency. Numerology leads to a melodic dance between you and the universe moving in flow and sensing sounds and tones of spirit's plan for you. It's an offering to let you know you always have a way to get back on track when you think you have detoured from your path.

Numerology offers us the tools to navigate the space we are currently inhabiting, guiding us through the winters and rainstorms (and sometimes hurricanes) of our life, but also preparing us for sunny days, to take advantage of the flowers in bloom and the quiet of winter, connecting us to those natural cycles of our lives.

I remember when I first truly understood what numerology was and how powerful it is. Even with my background in numbers, I wasn't familiar with the term *numerology* when I was growing up. I just knew that numbers had a spiritual meaning based off birthdays, addresses, phone numbers, and my grandmother winning money every week and Big Red pamphlets around her house and in her Bible.

When I first discovered numerology, I realized it is more than a metaphysical system that interprets the meaning and energies associated with numbers: It's also how the universe helps us understand life, personality traits, and our future destinies. Numerology is more than a practice stemming from ancient history; it's a poetic journey into the soul's language. I like to say it's a whisper from the universe keeping us on track. To some, numbers are just digits, but in the canyon, numbers are the breath of spirit speaking to the essence of our soul, allowing us to take in and accept the path we were meant to walk in this lifetime.

Each number carries a unique vibrational frequency that plays a specific part in each area of our life. Just like a paint-by-numbers picture, every number counts in the creation of a masterpiece. The numbers in our life paint a picture of our deepest selves, our challenges, and our potential. There are several numbers that you can paint a picture with in your life, but for the purposes of the canyon and the work you will continue to do, we'll be focusing on our life path, our personal year, and the universal year.

I have a saying that I teach to everyone I know when they are deciding how to use these three numbers during their journey in the canyon: The universal year is the season during your journey through the canyon, your personal year is the weather, and your life path is the wardrobe you wear along the way.

The universal year is the energy at play that applies to everyone globally. It's calculated by adding the digits of the current year.

(For example, 2025 is a 9: 2025 = 2 + 0 + 2 + 5 = 9.) This number sets the tone for the energies that everyone will experience during the year.

To some, these are just numbers, but these numbers have historical significance. Among the earliest known civilizations, the Sumerians in Mesopotamia used numbers primarily for admirative and economic purposes, such as record keeping, trade, and to allocate resources. They also associated numbers with spiritual symbolism, integrating them into their religious and cultural practices. Within Pythagorean mysticism, they established that numbers have distinct properties, which led them to believe that numbers play a crucial role in understanding the soul's journey and purpose. The Pythagoreans created the harmony of the spheres concept, which suggests that celestial bodies create forms of music and energies that are inaudible to the human ear but can be understood through numerical relationships. In a more contemporary example, Carl Jung explored the synchronicity of numbers and believed that numerical coincidences have deep spiritual significance. In our modern culture, numerology is still prevalent. Erykah Badu named her firstborn son Seven because, for her, the seventh letter of the alphabet, *G*, stands for god.

Every number holds a vibration that you carry with you throughout your lifetime. This is what keeps you in alignment as you journey through the canyon so you know you are moving in the right direction for an understanding of your soul's destiny. When in doubt, look to your numbers to help guide you through your own personal evolution. Your personal year, your life path, and the universal year allow you to stop forcing things. Whether around a relationship, job, or friendship, embodying alignment allows for ease. It can take away the hardness and rough edges in life. You get a chance to put yourself back on track at any point.

Your Life's Blueprint

LIFE CAN FEEL LIKE A MYSTERIOUS MAZE sometimes, as we search for direction, purpose, and a deeper understanding of ourselves. Ancient traditions have tapped these very questions, and numerology offers a unique lens through which to explore them. Imagine a world where numbers hold more than just quantitative value, where they vibrate with energy and whisper secrets about your life's journey. Numerology delves into this hidden language, revealing how the date you were born, your name, and even the current year all hold clues to your strengths, challenges, and the overall theme playing out in your life right now.

Think of yourself as a brave adventurer embarking on a grand quest. Numerology becomes your trusty map, pinpointing your life path, the core purpose that guides your entire journey. But the map is only the beginning. Each year brings a new season: a personal year number that influences the specific challenges and opportunities you'll encounter. Understanding these cycles allows you to navigate with more grace and awareness. And beyond your individual path, there's the universal year number, a collective energy affecting everyone that paints the broader landscape of the times we live in.

We all live within a nine-year cycle, where each year brings different energies and lessons. Master years, like 11, 22, and 33, can appear in your cycle and bring heightened experiences and spiritual growth. These master years can occur several times in your life or perhaps only once, depending on your unique numerological path.

Our personal year defines the themes and energies we'll experience throughout the year, while the universal year reflects the collective energy we all navigate. Personal years follow a nine-year cycle, each phase echoing similar lessons and themes.

Understanding both your personal year and universal year offers a comprehensive view of the influences shaping your journey. Your personal year number guides you through the unique challenges and opportunities you'll face each year.

Your life path number, like a wardrobe, evolves as you age—refining and adjusting to new experiences. For instance, if you're a life path 1, your innate leadership and self-starting qualities will transform over time, becoming more refined as you progress through different stages of life.

Numerology goes beyond simply calculating numbers. It's about understanding the energetic blueprint of your life and using that knowledge to live with more intention and purpose.

Embodying numerology becomes the act of recognizing any disharmony and weaving in the threads of healthy boundaries that are aligned with your personal numbers. It creates space for nurturing connections by going after opportunities and relationships that are in alignment with your core being. Embodying numerology isn't a rigid pursuit of perfection or coloring within the lines, but rather a continuous process of weaving your authentic self into the tapestry of your life. You can transform your understanding of numerology from a mere number to a vibrant and dynamic force guiding you toward your life purpose and fulfillment.

Numerology helps you make conscious choices and cultivate awareness based off your energetic blueprint, embodying the natural laws of the universe by letting you know that at your core, you are one with energies that make you you. You may believe that you were just born on a Tuesday, but the energy such information holds gives you the strength and tenacity to move through life to face challenges and to receive the abundance that spirit has to offer.

Your Magical Motherfucking Download

Ready to embark on this exciting exploration? The following exercises will guide you in calculating your life path and personal year numbers, offering a glimpse into the fascinating world of numerology and the valuable insights it holds for you.

Your Life Path—Your Wardrobe

To calculate your life path number, add your complete birth month, birthday, and birth year. For example, if you were born on January 11, 1989:

Add 1 + 1 + 1 + 1 + 9 + 8 + 9 = 30.

Then add those together: 3 + 0 = 3.

This birth date would be life path 3.

Note: If your final number is a double-digit master number (11, 22, 33), do not reduce it further. For instance, if the sum is 22, your life path number remains 22, not 2 + 2 = 4.

Each life path number corresponds to a set of characteristics that allow you to become deeply self-aware in recognizing your true calling by igniting your natural strengths. Your life path number provides you with insights into different phases of your life, helping you understand and navigate through the canyon. Here's how each life path helps you heal through the canyon:

Life path 1—The goal is to overcome issues that bring up self-doubt and codependency. When you have a life path 1, while you're in the canyon, trust in your ability to become independent.

Life path 2—The goal is to overcome any tendencies that allow you to become passive. You must develop emotional balance and know the difference between being supportive and being a martyr.

Life path 3—The goal is to narrow down your scattered energies and lack of discipline. When you are in the canyon, focus is the key. Deepen your emotional expression so you can learn how to become attached to the projects, people, and things that matter. This way, you'll be more inclined to take responsibility and not shy away from the commitments that are important to you.

Life path 4—The goal is to work on flexibility and being less allergic to change. When you become more adaptable and embrace change, being less rigid makes your journey through the canyon easier.

Life path 5—The goal is to not get attached to monotony. Discipline is important, but don't allow it to cloud your need to explore and embrace adventure while you create a more sensory experience in the canyon.

Life path 6—The goal is to not worry. Learn to balance being responsible and letting go at the same damn time. While you're in the canyon, do not be overly critical or interfere with your healing process.

Life path 7—The goal is to not isolate yourself. Trust others to contribute to your learning, as everyone has something to teach you. While in the canyon, balance your need to process what you are experiencing during your journey with periods of openness and connection, and call in the types of people you want to connect with.

Life path 8—The goal is to look beyond the material world and develop a deep sense of authenticity, because inner work is the true way to channel power, not external forces. While in the canyon, use your leadership abilities responsibly and ethically.

Life path 9—The goal is to balance any emotional ups and downs while you allow yourself to let go of the past. While in the canyon, develop forgiveness and unconditional love. Learn to let go of your past and move forward.

Life path 11—The goal is to overcome any fears or anxiety related to having high expectations for yourself. While in the canyon, trust your intuition and connect to spirit in the most practical ways.

Life path 22—The goal is to harness your potential to make a large impact. While in the canyon, you are meant to learn how to build solid foundations to use your abilities for the greater good.

Life path 33—The goal is balancing your personal life with the responsibilities of being a visionary. While in the canyon, you must learn how to heal and nurture others without sacrificing your personal happiness and joy.

Your Personal Year—The Weather

To calculate your personal year number, you will add your birth month and day and the current year. For example, if you were born on January 11, and it's 2025:

Add 1 + 1 + 1 + 2 + 0 + 2 + 5 = 12.

Then add those together: 1 + 2 = 3.

The personal year for this birthdate is 3.

Note: If your final number is a double-digit master number (11, 22, 33), do not reduce it further. For instance, if the sum is 22, your personal year number remains 22, not 2 + 2 = 4. In the realm of numerology, master numbers are highly spiritual and powerful numbers that carry a significant amount of potential and energy. Master numbers often indicate a greater level of responsibility and a stronger connection to spiritual and personal growth. When you encounter a master number in your personal year, it signifies a time of profound lessons and opportunities for enlightenment, building foundational work, or expressing visionary creativity. Embracing the energy of these master numbers can lead to a transformative period in your life, helping you achieve your higher purpose and impact the world around you.

This is the type of weather you can expect while you are traveling through the canyon:

Personal year 1—The energy that supports you during your time in the canyon is an energy of new beginnings. Your work in the canyon involves overcoming your fears of starting new ventures while addressing your self-doubt and self-worth.

Personal year 2—The energy that supports you during your time in the canyon is the energy of patience and partnership. Your work in the canyon requires you to address any issues of dependence.

Personal year 3—The energy that supports you during your time in the canyon is the energy of self-expression and joy. Your work in the canyon requires you to overcome your fears of being judged for your creative mind and learn to focus your scattered energies.

Personal year 4—The energy that supports you during your time in the canyon is the energy of stability and building a foundation. Your work in the canyon will challenge your resistance to structure and focus on creating personal rituals that allow you to incorporate disciplined routines that feel aligned.

Personal year 5—The energy that supports you during your time in the canyon is the energy of freedom and change. Your work in the canyon requires you to overcome your fears around change and learn to not cling to chaos.

Personal year 6—The energy that supports you during your time in the canyon is the energy of responsibility. Your work in the canyon is to foster solid relationships that provide an ebb and flow of giving and receiving nourishment for yourself, your family, and your home.

Personal year 7—The energy that supports you during your time in the canyon is the energy of inner work and spiritual growth. Your work in the canyon focuses on dealing with tendencies to detach from your inner child and past traumas. You must face them head-on.

Personal year 8—The energy that supports you during your time in the canyon is the energy of balancing personal achievement and material success. Your work in the canyon requires you to address any issues that make you lean toward material obsession and worldly power.

Personal year 9—The energy that supports you during your time in the canyon is the energy of reflection and completion. Your work in the canyon requires you to let go of the past and forgive yourself.

Personal year 11—The energy that supports you during your time in the canyon is the energy of spiritual enlightenment. Your work in the canyon requires you to address any anxiety that comes your way while dealing with an increased level of intuition.

Personal year 22—The energy that supports you during your time in the canyon is the energy of building something larger than life. Your work in the canyon requires you to face your fear of failure while also releasing yourself from high expectations.

Personal year 33—The energy that supports you during your time in the canyon is the energy of visionary creativity. Your work in the canyon involves balancing the wants and needs of others while tending to your personal life.

The Universal Year—The Season

To calculate the universal year number, you add each number of the current year. Remember that the universal year is something everyone will experience. For example, if the current year is 2025:

Add 2 + 0 + 2 + 5 = 9.

Thus 2025 is a universal year 9.

Here is the season that you will experience while traveling through the canyon:

Universal year 1—The season theme is learning to trust yourself.

Universal year 2—The season theme is finding an emotional equilibrium with relationships.

Universal year 3—The season theme is embracing creative talents and self-expression.

Universal year 4—The season theme is overcoming any fears about building a solid foundation.

Universal year 5—The season theme is embracing new experiences and balancing freedom and responsibility.

Universal year 6—The season theme is taking responsibility for your home and your family.

Universal year 7—The season theme is deepening your spiritual understanding within yourself.

Universal year 8—The season theme is stepping into your authority while cultivating values you can stick with.

Universal year 9—The season theme is about letting go of the past and forgiving yourself for past actions.

Universal year 11—The season theme is embracing your fear of the unknown and trusting your heightened intuition.

As you have likely seen from your own numerology and life, the path to alignment will not be a straight line. Each year will offer you valuable tools to understand your soul journey, revealing your core challenges and opportunities for growth. Understanding this can help you recognize any detours and guide you as you navigate your canyon, encouraging you to embrace flexibility and avoid clinging to the familiar.

Numerology allows you to release the past and align yourself with the energy that you are currently experiencing.

The Odyssey of Alignment

WHEN YOU EMBODY ALIGNMENT, IT CAN manifest in various ways. Your decision-making becomes more authentic, your actions are more congruent, and you are in harmony with your inner feelings and outer expressions. On an emotional level, alignment enhances your awareness and promotes balance and resilience. You can foster more authentic relationships with others and, most important, with yourself.

This work then becomes a deeply personal odyssey, demanding commitment to your self-discovery and a willingness to confront the depths of your inner landscape. Will this alignment process be challenging? Oh, hell yes, but it is also beautifully transformative.

In the canyon, you begin to untangle the intricate web of your past experiences by slowly releasing the heavy burdens and the conditioning that you've been taught. It might feel very delicate to unravel, but this process will allow you to reacquaint yourself with parts you've lost or have hidden away due to fear of judgment or shame. When you begin to align with your most authentic self and dance with the darkness of your soul, you can acknowledge your fears and stop suppressing your dreams. You begin to reshape who you are and integrate who you want to be. You begin to become whole.

Many of my friends and clients—and even myself—always reach out when they are at the precipice of their personal year 6. Personal year 6 can be a shit show. It's often considered the most challenging personal year in the cycle, but it can also be the most aligning. There is a lot of self-sacrifice and things you can't control during this year. At times, you find yourself constantly putting the needs of others before your own, putting out fires that you didn't start. Personal year 6 can make you become resentful and hinder your ability to care for yourself because it can feel like everything is beyond your control.

However, this year can also solidify the foundation of your life. It lays the groundwork for future happiness and abundance. This year teaches you how to advocate for yourself and communicate your needs more effectively. So even though this year feels like your world is falling apart, it's actually coming together. It is putting you on the true path of alignment.

Alignment helps you to not project your unresolved issues onto others, paving the way for more genuine and nourishing interactions. Alignment doesn't just become a personal victory, but it influences every relationship you cultivate.

Imagine you are the gardener of your life, tending to a garden that has been forgotten for years. You must be gentle while you are pulling up the withered plants. Think of those plants as parts of yourself that have been neglected over the years, and now you must spend time nurturing them and reviving them, giving them that attention and care that they once were denied. This healing is not just about removing the weeds of your past; it's about learning to see the beauty within that garden and appreciate what it is and what could be. You need courage for that. You need resilience for that. And resilience comes from being able to tend to the garden in the first place. When you begin to seek alignment in this part of the canyon, you begin to reclaim the parts of yourself that you've disowned or ignored. But when you integrate the essence of alignment, the wilted parts don't necessarily go away; they bring you closer to wholeness.

On the other hand, you can't run away from it when you're out of alignment. Things around you don't seem to go as well as you would like. Things will always feel forced if you continue pushing yourself, even when you don't feel like it at the moment. You've been taught that your life will take you on a path that is straight and uninterrupted. That sounds like the life of a robot: doing things that fit the status quo and being happy with whatever life has to offer. That is not alignment.

Getting aligned is about going on a journey with a destination in mind but knowing that you will get off track. It's inevitable that the road will change, and you may lose your map along the way. That's okay. What you need to understand is that being lost and out of alignment can be one of the best things to happen to you—not because you will feel good about it, but because you won't know you are off track until you start feeling that pull within. Getting aligned will allow you to keep promises to yourself that others broke throughout your life.

Healing the Wounds That Still Bleed

MY THERAPIST ONCE SAID TO ME, "We are all broken, but how we use our brokenness is what matters."

I truly thought that I would live with the feeling of brokenness

for the rest of my life, always feeling not worthy of goodness, or that I would always feel like I had to struggle. But that was false. What I needed to learn was how to take care of the younger version of myself in my adult body. Or as some say, I had to reparent myself. I needed to give myself what I needed when I was a four-year-old in the hospital alone night after night. I needed to comfort myself like I needed when I found out the truth about my biological father. I needed to tell myself the words of love that I needed when I suffered my first heartbreak. I had to start again but in a different way. I had to give myself the chance I never thought I had in life.

When I was younger, I would always overhear the man who raised me say, "She's been through a lot." As those words would come out of his mouth, I would agree but not truly acknowledge the "a lot" part. But once I started to go through my own canyon, I realized the magnitude of my life experiences and my upbringing. I don't blame anyone. If anything, my life lets me know that spirit hears me. Spirit hears all of us. My journey of healing has been complex and powerful not just for myself but for my lineage. The work that we do on ourselves not only heals us but also heals those who came before us and those who will come after. You may think working on yourself is just for you, but it's not.

Alignment lets us know these are the parameters that can help us become our best selves. If we can surrender to the parameters, we will have success and peace. If you are not willing to surrender, then you can become out of alignment with everything.

To connect with our alignment, we need to understand the natural cycles of our life path. Embodying alignment allows you to become your most authentic self by deeply connecting with your true feelings. This requires embracing your emotions rather than suppressing them. By honoring the natural rhythm of my emotions, I become my most authentic and psychic self. I reduce the friction between what I want and what I need to do, and I create a safe and harmonious environment within myself.

Alignment helps me form deeper relationships with others because I have love and understanding to give, having first given it to myself. It allows me to listen to what's calling me inside. When I get triggered by past events, I revisit what is bothering me and why I was triggered. This is spirit's signal that something within needs to be released. Alignment may not always be straight and narrow, but it offers an opportunity to be transparent with oneself, promoting a healthy relationship between mind and body.

Here are some questions to ask yourself when working on alignment:

1. What emotions arise when I reflect on my life path number?
2. How can I honor the natural rhythm of my emotions in my daily life?
3. In what ways can I reduce the friction between my desires and my actions?
4. How does my personal year number influence my current experiences?
5. What past triggers can I revisit to release unresolved feelings?
6. How can I create a safe, harmonious environment within myself?
7. What is my inner calling, and how can I align my actions with it?
8. How can I cultivate deeper relationships by first giving love and understanding to myself?

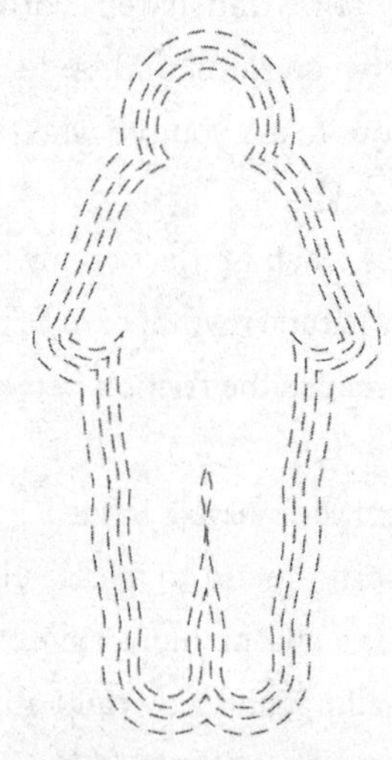

How Can I Connect to My Truth?

5

MEDIUMSHIP

The Embodiment of Truth

I BEGAN RUNNING FROM MY MEDIUMSHIP CAPABILITIES when I was a child—not because I was scared but because I didn't want to be different. There is something innocent about being oblivious to the spiritual world, especially when you can communicate with people who have crossed over. At one point in my life, I began to think being a medium was a burden—and who wants to live with the burden that has you tapped into the spirit realm all the time? I for sure didn't, but what I found over the years is that mediumship was my haven in this crazy world. I never felt alone, even as an only child in a big family, because I had a connection to the other side.

Whether it was the spirit guides I would talk to or the dreams I would have, I knew my ancestors and loved ones who passed were near and helping me in the physical world. I knew when people were about to die. When I worked in the corporate world, I gave a reading to a coworker at a seafood restaurant on our break. I saw a very clear vision of her father sitting in a recliner chair, his disability eating him alive. It was a very uncomfortable image. How was I supposed to relay this message? Should I keep it to myself?

When I was a baby psychic/medium I was reckless. I would shout, "Break up with him!" at friends. I would give unsolicited advice in the rawest way. That's how my guides communicated with me. I had to learn how to be quiet. I had to learn how to speak of death. So, I looked at my coworker and said, "Your dad is very sick. Do your best to make peace with him while you can." About a year later, she came back for another session and let me know that her dad had transitioned.

At first, I thought, *Well, at least I wasn't wrong.* As I began to understand why I was able to see death, I still resisted it. Why did I need to know when it was someone's time? I decided to leave mediumship behind because there was too much truth in it. It was too finite. I hadn't lived the life I wanted yet. There was so much more for me to experience, and I didn't want the cloud of death hanging over my life. I hadn't gotten married, had a child, bought a house, and so on. But to have to see dead people on top of all that? No, thank you. My mind was in shambles. I thought, *This is happening again. This mediumship is creeping in.* I just wanted to be intuitive and know a few things here and there to help people move forward. That's all.

This overwhelming feeling took me back to when my grandmother passed. The night before she passed, while my mother and

I were with her at the hospital, she called out to my grandfather, whom I'd never met. My heart sank and I sighed just a bit. I went home, and the next morning around four or five, the phone rang. I knew that was it. Many things led up to this loss. About two weeks or so before, I was getting ready to pledge a sorority when my body told me it wasn't the right time. I told the assistant dean of pledging that I couldn't do it. She told me that when the time was right to let her know. A week later, my grandmother passed. My body knew. My body always knows.

When the hospital called my mother and said Grandma was having complications, my mom rushed to the hospital. I took my time because I knew she was already gone. As I was leaving, my mom called back, and the only thing I heard on the other end of the phone was "She's gone." My mom was the youngest of eight. I could hear in her voice that her mommy was gone. I drove to the hospital and said goodbye as my grandmother's warm body laid there, her skin still moisturized from the day before. Afterward, my cousin and I drove to IHOP to get something to eat. On the radio, Boyz II Men's "A Song for Mama" started playing, and I cried as I drove.

A few nights later, I woke up to find my grandmother sitting on the edge of my bed. I wasn't sad or scared; I felt safe, and that let me know that she was with me. But it still didn't give me the urge to move toward my truth. I had the gift of mediumship, but I wanted to sugarcoat it as just being a psychic. That felt less weird and more on brand for me. Talking to people who had crossed over would make me weirder. So I tucked away my truth and went on with my life, but that never works. When you run from the truth, your truth finds you. It seeks you out like a needle in a haystack. There is a quote attributed to Mark Twain that has always stuck with me: "A lie can travel halfway around the world while the truth is putting on its shoes."

This means that the lies we tell ourselves or live by can spread quickly and gain momentum before we even realize it. These lies can influence our actions and beliefs, shaping our reality in ways that may not serve us. On the other hand, the truth often takes longer to surface. It's not because the truth is less powerful, but because it requires deeper introspection. Uncovering the truth involves peeling back layers of self-deception and facing uncomfortable realities. However, once the truth emerges, it brings clarity and alignment, allowing us to live more authentically.

The Mechanics of Mediumship

TO SOME, MEDIUMSHIP FEELS LIKE MAGIC, but in essence it is an acknowledgment of the spiritual realm without bias and an understanding that there is more to this life than living in the physical world. Mediumship in its most sacred form is not just communicating with the dead. It is a journey toward the core of our truth, of our being in human form. The bridge between our personal truths and where our ancestors reside may seem like a bridge that spans a million miles, but it's closer than we think. The veil is very thin.

To embody truth through mediumship, you must remember that truth is not a destination. It is a process toward understanding not only ourselves but our connection to the universe, to spirit. Mediumship becomes somewhat of a mirror that reflects the many dimensions of our existence. It presents us with an opportunity not only to confront our present but also to shine a light on the shadows of our past. It speaks something that has been unspoken about those who have come before us and those who are presently with us. When we dialogue with those who have departed, we are given a chance that transcends time and space and that aligns us with our lineage.

Ancestral voices that are often silenced by our everyday lives and capitalistic goals are allowed to come forth and reveal to us the truth of our ancestral stories, which can invoke hope, love, and resilience, and not just fear of death. It was the fear of death and the unknown that held us back, creating barriers to understanding our true selves and our purpose. By embracing these ancestral truths, we move beyond the fear that once paralyzed us, allowing for a more profound connection to our heritage and a clearer path forward. It lets us know that we are a part of a larger narrative that extends beyond our human experience and beyond what we can see with our mind's eye. In this space of the unseen, our truths begin to crystalize, becoming tangible. We begin to understand the patterns and cycles of our families. We begin to understand the unhealed wounds that have subconsciously shaped us.

When we are ready for this truth, its awareness is game-changing because it not only allows us to heal ourselves, but it heals everyone around us and those who might come after us. You may believe that your healing is just for you, but it's more than you. It's more than you and more than me; it's for the greater good of the community, whether the community you've chosen or the one you were born into, now and on into the future. Mediumship guides us and nurtures us into our most authentic selves. It teaches us to trust our souls and listen to the wisdom that our ancestors have to offer us. When we listen to our ancestors, we can live a more aligned life—a life that continues to put us on the path of our deepest truths.

Mediumship is a sacred dance with the invisible, a dance that invites us to embrace the full spectrum of our existence. It allows us to explore what is beyond the veil, and through this exploration, we come to embody our truth—not as a static entity, but as a living, breathing, eternal essence that evolves with each step we take on this eternal journey of self-discovery and spiritual awakening.

Mediumship provides us a unique way of healing because what we most need and desire in the physical world is connection to the memories that allow us to feel real love, real hope. When someone you love passes on to the other side, you miss them because you can no longer create memories with them; you know they won't be part of your future. Mediumship offers us a connection to what we may have lost in the physical world. We experience pain and sadness once someone has passed on, and we tend to forget the truth of what they showed us or what we experienced with them while they were here. When you communicate with spirits, you receive guidance to help you understand your family's truths and legacy. You not only get personal revelations and insights, but you get confirmation about yourself and your life circumstances, along with the familiar comfort of connecting with a loved one.

Our ancestors guide us in the most miraculous ways. My grandmother would tell me stories about how her loved ones from the other side would speak to her in her dreams, giving her guidance about what to do in the present. When I started having dreams about my departed relatives and visions about future events, she knew I had a connection to the spirit realm that was unique, and she nourished it both while on earth and after she transitioned.

My connection to her continues to support me in everything I do. I have less fear of the spirit world, and I feel more confident when I give readings and work with clients; she has shown me how to be a clear vessel for spirit.

What begins to happen when we can embody truth? We embrace the flow of our lives, accepting the best and worst parts of ourselves and giving ourselves permission to exist in our fullness. We stop pretending. Instead, we get comfortable in our skin, allowing every part of ourselves to be seen. We find comfort in the unknown because all that matters is the present, and we are deep enough into our healing now to know that all we can shape is the present. We have gone into the canyons of our souls, and we have been willing not only to see the truth of our past, our path, our choices, and our visions but to embrace all of it.

The Big Leap

MY FIRST MEDIUMSHIP MENTOR WAS an older eastern European woman. She was tiny, had curly salt-and-pepper hair, and would host mediumship development classes in her home with small groups. I'd contemplated taking her classes for years because I knew I had the talent and gift of mediumship, but I wasn't ready to explore it. I knew about her through peers who had taken her classes before. I didn't want to activate the dead coming to visit me, just as they had done at night when I was in high school and college.

Back then, when my mediumship and psychic ability was loud and in color, it caused me to begin using over-the-counter sleep medication just to get a good night's sleep. It started with one Benadryl a night, but by the time I was in college, I was on two and a half nighttime ibuprofen, causing me to become dependent on over-the-counter sleep medications. This was all so I didn't have visitors or dreams because I wanted that freedom to just be. Eventually, my mom intervened and made me realize that I could be damaging my liver. I stopped cold turkey and never looked back. After this, finding sleep was a challenge that I never expected. I learned how to heal my lack of sleep by taking classes on aromatherapy and creating tinctures and a better sleep atmosphere for myself by wearing an eye mask and turning off my phone.

Taking this class was a big leap back into mediumship, but I deeply felt spirit calling me to it. I registered and the instructor started the course by offering the group snacks and a variety of teas. One tea I had never tried was calling me: Bengal Spice by Celestial Seasonings. This brand of tea was the one that I burned myself with when I was four, but the flavor then was Sleepytime. A warm feeling washed over my body, and I made a cup for myself. I sipped the tea, and the class began a meditation.

Our teacher explained that we would feel the temperature in the room drop at some point, and that was a clear indication that spirit was present. We began to give readings to one another, and I had a chance to read for her. What I was shown was magical, and it was hard for me to comprehend because it was unfamiliar. Her parents came through; she confirmed what I was seeing, and I wasn't shocked. But I was a little angry. For so long, I thought my talent of connecting to people on the other side would make me weird. I came to realize my power in that moment, and I couldn't help but feel a little heartbroken.

I knew this was my calling, even though a part of me didn't want it. I didn't resonate with any of the psychics or mediums that I had seen on the internet or on TV. This teacher stood out to me because she taught me that mediumship is different for everyone. Some people actually see the spirits physically; some feel them, and some see them just in their mind's eye. Once again, I put it to the side and said, *If it's meant to be, it will come back to me.*

Mediumship

Death and I have a very interesting relationship. It might start with a knowing that I sense and feel in someone's spirit, or perhaps someone's loved one comes through when I am just sitting next to them; that can haunt me. I truly don't like knowing this information, but time and time again, when I am forced, often unwillingly, to enter my canyon, I recognize that this is part of the work I've come here to do: to guide, teach, and bridge the material world and the spiritual. I am here to take two concepts and combine them to make others understand how difficult information—the truth—can help them heal.

The work that I do isn't just about acknowledging trauma; it's about alchemizing it. When it seems like all is lost, there is always something out there to learn, and that's how I use mediumship to guide me and the people I work with. I look at the blessing of being able to connect with my ancestors as a gift to create, to live whole in a fragmented world. That is how we alchemize pain into purpose—we look for the missing pieces, and we create something entirely new. It takes courage to create something new, especially when being different isn't appreciated until you prove it works or that it's a better way.

Mediumship may feel like an extraordinary journey, but it's something most of us do daily. You may not be a professional medium, like me, and that is just fine. And quite frankly, for the purposes of this journey through the canyon, you only need to scratch the surface. Opening yourself up to mediumship is not just about connecting with spirits or your ancestors; it's about achieving a deep understanding of yourself. When you begin to travel through this part of the canyon, you are ready to cultivate a concrete foundation of self-awareness. This can be accessed in various ways, and I especially like meditation to open a channel.

The first step in any spirit communication is to set a clear intention that you want to connect with a loved one or ancestor. Many people are surprised how far a clear intention can go when it comes to communicating with spirit. In many cases, we don't get what we want when we ask spirit for things, which is because we haven't set a clear intention. Spirit doesn't like confusion; spirit operates through clarity and intention. Your intention serves as a guiding light throughout your journey through the canyon. Remember you are already psychic, but you may not have the heighted sense of awareness you once had as a child or a baby, because you've been accumulating trauma, conditioning, and other barriers that cause you to not hear spirit well.

As you are developing your psychic abilities, it's time to tap in and pay attention to your instincts and dreams and the subtle energies that have been guiding you all along. Now you are ready to hear them and feel them because your heart, mind, and body have the capability to experience the truth. I know you've heard the saying "The truth will set you free," but the truth can only do that if you intend or want to be free. And only if your body can handle it.

Most of our journey focuses on the mind, which is great and helps us, but the body doesn't lie. The body holds your truth. The body knows when it's ready to experience something and when it's ready to run. In this part of the canyon, you are ready to hear the truth and connect with it. You are ready to practice trusting spirit and your loved ones who have crossed over. They are always trying to communicate with you, but unfortunately, you've been conditioned to not hear them.

As you begin to build a relationship with mediumship, a sacred space is crucial. This can be a physical or mental space that makes you feel safe to do spiritual work. This space must be sacred, you must protect it and ensure that you energetically keep that space and yourself safe. When you tap into the skill of mediumship, remember that patience, practice, and perseverance are key to developing the connection. While you are in the canyon, you will practice understanding mediumship for the purpose of connecting to your truth. As you build a strong relationship with your loved ones, what you hear, see, and smell are more than just messages. They become a reflection of your own life, emotions, and spiritual path. Mediumship brings you insight into your own nature and life choices, and it shows you that we are all interconnected. This journey is not just about connecting with spirits; it's also about deepening your understanding of yourself and the universe around you.

Digging Deep into Self-Awareness

THE ONE THING I HAVE LEARNED about canyon work is that you can't get out until you've been willing to dig deep. And through mediumship, we start by building a strong foundation of self-awareness.

This part of the canyon encourages you to tap into your instincts, dreams, and subtle energies. When life throws up a lot of noise, mediumship teaches you to quiet your mind and listen. Your body often holds on to unprocessed emotions and experiences. This part of the canyon emphasizes tuning in to your body's signals to understand your readiness to hear your guides or your ancestors.

Mediumship connects us to our truth because when we start or get deeper into the healing journey, we will want to know if we're on the right path. Going into those canyons alone can be terrifying—there's a reason we avoided them for this long—but when you begin to build a relationship with your guides, they will not only offer you signs along the path, leading you to where you want to go, they will provide love and comfort, and the deep wisdom that has been in you all along. When you are in the psychical world, you often question the meaning of life, especially your life. Someone is listening, and that is spirit. I often test spirit in various ways to show me that what I am hearing and seeing is real.

Spirit always answers. My ancestors always answer. It amazes me that for so long I doubted my connection to source because society made me believe that my connection had to be a spectacle and that I couldn't naturally be with these gifts and talents and live my everyday life. I ran away from my gifts for so long to appease capitalist views on what was acceptable as a career and what was not. I was ashamed to say I was a psychic and medium. I was running away from my truth. "You can run, but you can't hide" is an age-old adage that tells us no matter how far you run away from your problems, passions, or purpose, you can't hide from them.

You get the opportunity to connect to your truth, and that connection births the most authentic version of yourself.

That's exactly why connecting to your truth through the lens of mediumship is important. Your ancestors don't lie. They have no reason to lie in the afterlife. On earth they may have told a few little lies here and there or maybe even a few big ones, but on the other side they offer you truth. They offer you a reason to believe that you aren't alone in this world. I know it's hard to fathom that while you are healing and growing through the motions on earth that your ancestors are right there with you, but they are. I feel protected when I ask my ancestors to give me the truth. Your ancestors want to communicate with you to help you heal, and they do this by showing you symbols, giving you feelings, or using other subtle forms of communication. Spirit doesn't waste time. There are no coincidences. It's important for you to be open to the messages that you will receive and the experiences that you will have once you get comfortable with your ancestral connections.

A Brief History of Mediumship

MEDIUMSHIP IS THE PRACTICE OF mediating communication between familiar spirits or spirits of the dead and living human beings. There are many types of mediums, but the most common are known as spirit mediums. Some people might even classify spirit channeling as mediumship, but it's not.

In tribal cultures, communicating with spirits has long been present in various forms. Shamanism, for example, involves a priest or priestess reaching an altered state of consciousness to interact with the spirit world. Shamanism is considered a precursor to modern mediumship. In tribal cultures, people would go see the shaman for various things that included healing as well as communicating with ancestors.

Many African societies have a longstanding spiritual tradition involving communication with ancestors and the spirit world. These practices involve ritualistic ceremonies and spiritual elders who communicate between the physical and the spiritual realms—another precursor to mediumship. During the transatlantic slave trade, also known as the Middle Passage, many of the slaves brought to America were forced to let go of their spiritual practices to follow the religion of their captors. African spiritual practices merged with Indigenous, European, and Christian beliefs, forming different syncretic religions.

Religious syncretism is the blending of two or more religious belief systems into a new system or the incorporation of other beliefs into an existing religious tradition. These are the origins of Voodoo in Haiti, Santeria in Cuba, Candomblé in Brazil, and Hoodoo in the southern United States. In these syncretic religions, spiritual leaders, such as priests and priestesses—houngans and mambos in Voodoo and Babalawos and Santeras in Santeria—have played a role like mediums, acting as bridges to the spiritual and physical worlds.

The mid-nineteenth century saw the birth of the Spiritualism movement, started by the Fox sisters in Hydesville, New York, who held séances and were known to communicate with spirits. Spiritualism quickly spread from the United States to Europe and became extremely popular in the United Kingdom. Magician Harry Houdini and members of the American Society for Psychical Research did extensive investigations of mediums, and although they exposed many frauds, they discovered that mediumship was real among a select few.

Carl Jung, the famed psychologist, also explored the realm of the medium. Jung's interest in the unconscious mind and the collective unconscious led him to believe in the potential validity of certain psychic phenomena. His work helped broaden the study of mediumship, suggesting that these experiences could reveal deeper truths about the human psyche.

During the nineteenth-century Spiritualism movement, there was a strong focus on communication with the dead through mediums. Mediums and psychics had a significant impact on the Black community, primarily through the church, where they were often referred to as prophets. It has been said that many leaders in the

Black community *had the gift*, which is what they said about certain people in the South.

It was known that Harriet Tubman used spells to free over 750 slaves and was able to do so because of her relationship with god/spirit. She knew which way to travel north, and it was even known that she could predict events before they occurred.

In Martin Luther King's March on Washington speech, he said he had a dream. In Southern culture, dreaming is linked to talking to ancestors and getting visions about the future and the past. His dream called for equality for all. In the Black community, the spiritual practitioners who were linked to the church were also community leaders, healers, and sources of guidance in times of oppression and social turmoil. Black and Caribbean cultures have learned to use mediumship and spirit communication as a therapeutic means to cope with trauma, keep cultural identity, and foster community.

My grandmother was a member of St. Catherine of Sienna, the Catholic church in St. Albans, New York, as well as Unity Church. She had an at-home daycare where she raised three generations of the church community. She was also a healer. When she would go to the Church of Unity retreats, doctors would ask her about her at-home remedies, which helped heal her children and the children she would look after. These are things that came to her from the spirit world as well as her ancestors in the South. In the present day, mediums are popular because they not only help people connect to their loved ones but also provide a gateway to healing. This is a pivotal moment when intuition begins to show up and the work you have been doing begins to manifest in the choices you are making in your life, understanding what has happened to you, and embracing the truths of your life. You become the voice of truth because you can hear those ancient guides within you.

Your Magical Motherfucking Download

The offering here is holding space for your ancestors through altar creation and spending time with them. Ask them questions and build the relationship. We think we're alone, but we are not. In this chapter, I offer practices to teach you how to lean in to these relationships. The more you practice, the easier it will be to start asking questions and listening to what your ancestors have to say.

An Altar to Invite Our Guides

I'VE USED MEDIUMSHIP TO EMBODY TRUTH by being open to what my ancestors wanted to say to me and guide me through, but some messages I couldn't receive until I could go deeper into my healing journey. I have done this in many ways, but one of my favorite ways is creating an altar and spending time with my ancestors. I have been able to build strong relationships with my guides, who have helped me root myself in my healing. There have been days when I didn't know if I would make it, or if there was anything to live for, and through my connection with my ancestors, I've been able to seek guidance to keep going.

The practices that I have cultivated with my spiritual team have helped me center myself and call on my ancestors when I need them most. The practice of building an altar and communing with ancestors can be a powerful component of spiritual growth and self-development. An ancestor altar serves as a sacred space where you can dedicate and honor your relationship with spirit to support your journey through the canyon. It represents a physical connection to your lineage and heritage. Common items to feature on an altar can include photographs, candles, incense, flowers, and personal mementos.

When it comes to altars, I like to make sure that all the elements are represented: water, earth, air, and fire. For water, I get a nice glass that would represent my loved one. My grandmother loved crystal glassware, so I have a very fancy piece of glass that sparkles in the candlelight. I fill it with water daily. For earth, I love flowers or dirt or anything that represents earth for your ancestor. Air is represented by the smoke rising from candles, and the flame represents fire.

Altars also include offerings such as food, certain drinks, and items that were significant to your ancestors when they were alive. Your altar should be in a place that is quiet and shows respect to your ancestors. I like to keep my altar in my room; some people have a special corner for theirs. I suggest you put yours where you feel most comfortable and where the energy feels peaceful.

After you build your altar, it's time to build a relationship with your ancestors. Visiting and talking to your ancestors daily is very important. I visit and talk to my ancestors daily. I start my day with them, and I end my day with them. You have permission to do what feels right to you. The time you spend with your ancestors in silence prepares you to hear from them. You may think that they are far away, but as I've stated before, the veil is thin, and the more you build your connection with them, the easier it will be to hear them.

When you ask questions to seek guidance from your ancestors through mediumship, be clear about the questions. You must also be open to receiving answers to these questions in various ways. You can receive answers through intuitive thought, through your dreams, or through signs and symbols in your daily life.

The only caveat about being in this part of the canyon is that

the truth may take a little bit longer for you to receive clarity and communication from your spirit team. This period requires patience and trust for the messages to unfold at the right time. During this part of healing, you are at somewhat of a crossroads because one part of you has healed and another part of you may not be ready for the truth. You must be ready to accept what spirit sends you. This takes patience and time with feeling, listening, and seeing. At first, it might feel like a fantasy, but pure intention and trust in the process are required. Embrace the journey with an open heart and mind, knowing that the truth will reveal itself in time.

Here are a few questions that I suggest asking when you are in this part of the canyon:

1. What lessons from your life can help me grow as a person?
2. How can I better understand my purpose and path in life?
3. What guidance can you offer me about strengthening my relationship with _____?
4. How can I break generational curses to benefit anyone who comes after me?
5. What career path or life pursuits would align with my true self?
6. How can I overcome the obstacles I'm currently facing in my business or professional life?
7. How can I deepen my spiritual practice and my connection to spirit/god?
8. What can I do to find peace and balance in times of stress or turmoil?
9. What are the most important values and lessons from our family history that I should carry forward?
10. How can I honor and continue your legacy in my daily life?
11. What insight can you provide about the important decisions I'm facing?
12. How can I recognize and follow the best path for my life journey?

13. How can I approach healing from both physical and emotional pain?
14. What ancestral remedies or practices might benefit my health and well-being?
15. How can I forgive those who have wronged me?
16. Is there anything in our family history that needs forgiveness or reconciliation?
17. What steps should I take to achieve my dreams and aspirations?
18. How can I stay motivated and focused on my goals?
19. What aspects of our heritage are important for me to learn and preserve?
20. Can you provide me with insights into our family's history and its impact on who I am?

After you pick your question or questions, it's time to listen and observe. This is where things can get tricky. Building your relationship with your ancestors is more about listening than speaking. It's important to pay attention to any feelings, thoughts, or sensations that arise during your time at the altar or when they begin to send you messages. While you are in the canyon, one of the practices that you can do to continue to build your relationship is meditation, which will help you increase your sensitivity to the spiritual realm.

Keeping a journal for your dreams is key. You might receive messages through your dreams, or you might have different thoughts and experiences while you sleep that you want to interpret. Building a relationship with your ancestors is a personal and unique journey that will take time, but the benefits you gain from the connection will support your healing. The key to doing this work in this part of the canyon is consistency, openness, and respect for your connection to building a relationship with your ancestors.

When you open up to this level of work, you open a channel for wisdom, guidance, and a deeper understanding of both you and the larger forces that are at play in your life. You will align with your spirituality, and it will transcend the physical.

Sacred Truths

I HAVE A UNIQUE RELATIONSHIP with mediumship. One part of me is always open to hearing what spirit has to say, and another part of me doesn't want to listen. On our journey in the canyon, asking the question *How can I connect to my truth?* can be one of the hardest embodiments to embrace, learn from, and listen to. The truth can be heartbreaking. The truth can be painful in the moments when we want other things to happen or other answers from our spirit team.

When we ask for the truth, we must be prepared for what the truth can offer us and how we will move forward with that truth. When spirit tells you that it's time to let go of a friendship or end an intense romance that's unhealthy for your growth, you must do it. Sometimes you don't, and you face the repercussions of not listening to what your ancestors have to say.

I often receive guidance in my dreams or through meditation at my altar. If you are wondering what the difference is between channeling and mediumship, I want you to think about listening to the radio. Just as each radio station has its own frequency, the frequency for human mediumship is lower than the frequency for channeling your guides and/or higher self. This is why I can't emphasize enough that while you are in this part of the canyon, the veil is thin and your ancestors are closer than you think.

Mediumship

After the pandemic, I was feeling very uneasy where I was. I had a products-based business that turned my apartment into a factory, and after I decided to shut down that business, I felt like my time where I was living had come to an end. I felt it in my body, which began to feel uneasy. Nights of good sleep were few and far between. I did what I knew I had to do when I was at a crossroads and needed answers: I called on my grandmother. The relationship that she and I have is a very sacred one. When I need her, there are several ways that I call on her. One of them is through my dreams, when I ask her to come and visit me.

So, before I went to bed one night, I stood at my altar and began to ask the questions I needed to ask. Should I move, and where should I go? I went to sleep, and like clockwork, she came to me around the time I was born, and I felt a pressure of someone sitting on the edge of my bed, and I woke up and saw a glimpse of her in a black-and-white striped shirt she wore, and I felt her voice saying it was okay to move, and I'll know the place because it will be easy.

The next morning, as I was doing my skin-care routine, I knew where I was headed next, and I knew that I would be there to connect with my ancestral roots even deeper and create something major in my life. I knew I'd be writing this book before it was ever set in stone. I chose my place, and she was right: It was easy. Within six weeks, I was on my way to a new city. During that move, many things were brought to light about my trust in the unknown. The truth is unknown because it is unbiased. It doesn't take sides; it simply provides exactly what you need. But we must listen to what the truth is saying, or we miss its message, its lesson, and its blessing.

Our guides are patient, but ultimately, we must show up. When my grandmother died, my mediumship truly opened. It was almost like she was waiting to get to the other side to show me more of my gifts. My dreams got deeper, more vivid. I was able to go back in time and astral travel and see things that I had never seen before. That was a truth that I wasn't ready for, but that truth was waiting for me. It was a truth that I needed to embrace with open arms and take seriously. There are many truths that you haven't embraced, that you've been ignoring due to fear. It's time to realize that the truth offers you a life that is filled with your soul's promise.

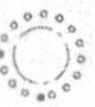

MEDIUMSHIP OFFERS US A PROFOUND PERSPECTIVE when we desire to know the greater truths of ourselves and the world around us. Our souls survive our physical death, and that gives us the ability to connect with the consciousness of our ancestors who have passed on. When you are open to mediumship, you gain insights into the nature of existence, the continuity of life, and the connection to all beings, both physical and nonphysical. Mediumship challenges you to expand your understanding of reality and consciousness. You may view the material world as the only world, because of course you have to live in it, and capitalism has done its best to make sure you live in a way that only honors what you can see right in front of your face. But the material world is just one small aspect of a much larger multidimensional universe.

My grandmother used to say, "But who are they in the spirit world?" We can get caught up with status and material things like cars, houses, and trips, but as my grandmother used to say, the devil wants you to be mesmerized by false prophets, but who is that person in the spiritual world? What is the truth of their soul? "A soul will reveal itself, if you just give it time," my grandmother would say. And that's the only version of that person's truth you need to be concerned with: Is there soul? This is the reason why, as a child, if I was uncomfortable with someone, my family and friends would take heed. It's as if they knew on some level that my awareness of the spirit world was heightened. I know my grandmother believed this.

When you make the decision in the canyon to tap into your mediumship, you are able to tap into other realms, and that creates a sense of security to help you understand that your perception of your reality is a small part of a much bigger and more complex tapestry of your soul and its existence. Your reality is more intertwined and less linear than your everyday experiences offer you. Mediumship provides comfort and healing and the knowledge that you are always in the presence of your loved ones, whether you feel it or not. It brings solace to your grieving heart, and it reinforces the belief that death is not an end but a sacred transition to another state of being. When you can accept that there is another state of being beyond just the physical, you can travel through your canyon with more grace and ease, ultimately discovering deeper truths, uncovering treasures beyond your wildest dreams, and experiencing a journey filled with extraordinary revelations.

No, this doesn't take away the heartache and pure agony of journeying through the canyon, but it provides you with an understanding that mortality is just one phase of your soul's journey. You develop a deeper appreciation for the continuity of life and know that you can get through every challenge that you are presented with. When you connect to loving spirits, you will receive messages of love and forgiveness and, most important, the ability to resolve unfinished emotional business that may be weighing you down in your present life. You get an opportunity to live more fully and authentically now and not wait for the future.

Mediumship inspires spiritual growth and development. When

you tap into this part of the canyon, you get a renewed sense of purpose and a deeper understanding of your spiritual journey and why it's important for you to carry on. The insights that you can gain from mediumship can lead to new possibilities of personal values, beliefs, and priorities that catalyze significant life changes and give you a greater sense of empathy for yourself and others. Now don't get me wrong. Connecting to mediumship during this part of the canyon doesn't loosen up your boundaries—it makes them stronger.

Because I do this work professionally, my boundaries have strengthened, knowing that everyone gets the opportunity to build a connection with spirit and develop strengths to heal themselves just like I have. When you open yourself to the greater truths of the universe and question the material world, you invite the mysteries of spiritual dimensions to change your view of the world. In a world where we only see materialistic perspectives, mediumship provides a perspective that emphasizes the importance of the spiritual world. Pathways are opened, and it challenges our conventional views of reality, providing healing and comfort.

Mediumship offers us a level of truth that we can't see. The healing journey in the canyon begins to get rough at this point. If you want to know your soul's truths, you can't move forward in your healing journey without building a relationship with your ancestors, especially the ones who watch over and protect you. This allows you to shift perspectives, challenge the status quo, and accept the possibility that there is more to existence than what we see in the physical realm. This mental shift is important while you travel through the canyon because you and your soul are cocreating your existence in the physical world with the help of insights from the spiritual world.

When you begin to incorporate their insights, you gain so

much from the relationship you build with your ancestors. You might rethink your beliefs about life, death, and the pure nature of consciousness. Your personal worldview begins to foster emotional healing and spiritual growth beyond the surface. It brings you a sense of peace and an appreciation for how you are being supported in other realms. The lessons that you learn from mediumship manifest in profound ways that change your self-concept and give you an increased sense of empathy and an appreciation for the present.

With an understanding that the present is a gift, you can get closer to your soul, closer to your most authentic self. You become deeply moved by your experiences with your ancestors, and you broaden your horizons to be a support for others. Ultimately, exploring these realms shapes your journey as well.

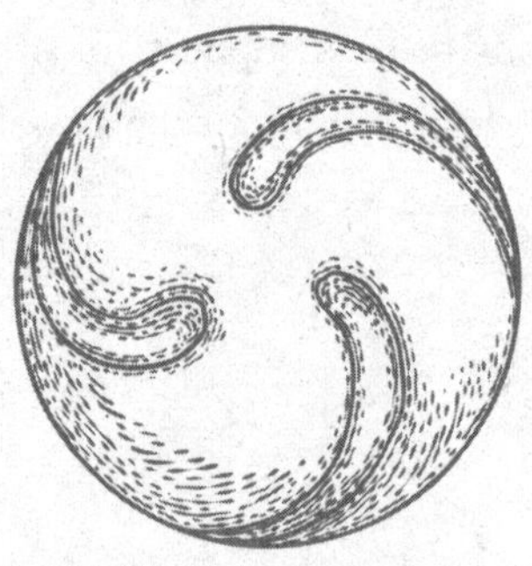

Why Am I Choosing This Life?

6

METAPHYSICS

The Embodiment of Choice

AS YOU READ THIS CHAPTER, I have a very clear disclaimer that I want you to take in as you enter this part of the canyon: You cannot manifest your way out of poverty. That is a complete lie. Poverty and systematic oppression are not things that you can eliminate by waving a magic wand. You can, however, manifest opportunities to get yourself out of poverty.

My background is a mix of middle class and upper middle class, fueled by a drug dealer with a college degree. Weed was the drug, and in the 1980s and '90s, it was illegal. Today, weed has been legalized in several states and has created many multimillionaires. The sale of it is considered a cool job where privileged white men have been able to utilize the system to their benefit and profit off something that has put many Black and Brown people in prison for years. The weed industry was shunned when it didn't benefit white men, but now it's glorified and an actual career field of choice, with colleges and business classes to help you maximize profit and do it the legal way. But many of the Black and Brown men and women with weed violations on their records cannot participate in this economic system. And my father is one of them.

I share this to point out that something that grows from our earth has been used to tear apart many families and communities. During the 1980s and '90s, it exposed me to a way of life that many haven't experienced. Now, I grapple with the internal struggle that what I once felt ashamed of is today the norm for many.

But because of my upbringing and the man who raised me, I learned the major lessons about choice. I learned the biggest lessons about creating your own destiny in a world where society will do anything to keep you down. This upbringing, though rough and complex, is what molded my tenacious ability to see the bright side in everything and see the world's possibilities even when my back is against the wall. This life gave me my grit, my femininity, and my grace, and it opened my eyes to my destiny. This life taught me what choice really is. And that's what your life has given you.

When you enter this part of the canyon, know that you may feel the urge to stop what you are doing and evaluate your next steps, which is fine. But remember this: You were dealt a set of cards when you entered this life, and those are the only cards you get. You can't exchange them, but what you can do is play them. You can play the hand that spirit/god has dealt you, and you can win at your own game. I want to teach you how to play the hand you've been dealt. I want to show you how to gracefully win against all odds.

Metaphysics

I will never forget the first time I watched the documentary called *The Secret,* and obviously I wasn't alone. An entire generation was introduced to metaphysics through *The Secret*—along with *What the Bleep Do We Know!?*—which showed us the science behind the energy we couldn't see but could feel was there. The core of *The Secret* is the law of attraction, which essentially states that like attracts like. This means that the energy and thoughts we put out into the universe have a direct impact on what we attract into our life.

Positive thoughts and intentions can bring about positive outcomes, while negative thoughts can attract negative experiences. Energy work became a powerful tool during this era, as people started to realize that the vibrations we emit don't just stay within us. They ripple out across everything we touch, think, and feel. What the eye can't see, energy can. It's that invisible force that's always there, whether we want to acknowledge it or not. It's the silent puppet master, pulling the strings behind the scenes, linking our thoughts to our reality in ways that can feel unbelievable until you start believing it. This is why energy work hit a nerve with so many people. It wasn't just some fluffy, feel-good concept. It was a way to take control of the unseen shit that runs our lives, to bend the currents and make the universe bend back. When you strip it all down, that's what we were all craving—something real, something raw, something that gives us the power to shape our world from the inside out.

The science behind this energy involves our understanding of quantum physics and the power of our minds. Quantum physics suggests that everything in the universe is made up of energy and that our thoughts and feelings are forms of energy as well. When we focus our minds on certain outcomes, we can influence the energy around us, essentially creating our reality through our intentions and beliefs. And what we discovered was that we could also participate in that energy, guiding elements of our lives and choosing how we react to the challenges of living.

I was taught the secret way before I ever saw the documentary. When my father would drive me to school, he would say to me, "The world is yours" and "You can have anything you want if you just put your mind to it." I believed him, but I wasn't quite sure if that was true for me. I grew up in a family where on my mother's side—which I was the closest to—I was the darkest one. I was told by cousins that my mom found me in a trash can, and in school I was compared to my lighter-skinned friends. I always felt ugly.

My dad never called me pretty or beautiful—not because I wasn't but because he wanted me to know I was smart and intelligent. That I was sure of very quickly. I was brown, with kinky curly hair, and I had a burn scar on my arm. I was different, and I knew that difference was going to be my advantage. What would make me stand out from the crowd? The answer for me, at first, was fashion. As I started getting older, I turned to fashion as a means of rebellion. *Even if the boys don't pick me first because I'm brown, at least I'm fly.* Fashion was my saving grace, and because I used it as a tool and almost as a weapon, I was able to change my self-concept without even knowing.

When I watched *The Secret*, I was intrigued but I was also confused. *So I could just change my mind about something, then the world would respond? That doesn't even make sense*, I thought to myself, and just a few short months after that, I understood why. There is no way it's that easy to just think a thought and then—bam!—your life has changed. So, I did what I knew best and went to Barnes & Noble and started looking at books on trauma. I came across so many books, and as I glanced through them, I received a download from spirit. I heard spirit say, *You must feel it in your body to believe it*. And then it all made sense.

My manifestations and self-concept didn't change in what I thought was my ugly era or because I said *I'm beautiful* in the mirror every morning before I got on the high school bus. No, it was because I felt it. When I put on a new outfit or put together some unique color combination, I felt good, I felt attractive, I felt unstoppable, and I felt pretty. This led me to understand that the secret does work, but it's different for people with complex trauma. The secret opened my eyes to creating a new world and playing a different game with the cards I had been dealt, but it also confirmed that creation would be different for me because I had so much trauma stored in my body that my brain just couldn't affirm my way out of it. Manifestation is a powerful tool, but for those raised by emotionally immature or toxic parents, it's a different ball game. Early experiences shape our core beliefs and energy, creating subconscious blocks that can seriously hinder our ability to manifest our deepest desires.

Growing up with an emotionally immature parent was incredibly confusing. Constantly being told I was selfish, being called names, and having to walk on eggshells made it hard for me to believe in my own thoughts and feelings. The very person who was supposed to believe in me and lift me up made me feel like she didn't even like me. This created deep feelings of unworthiness, fear, and self-doubt.

Let's be clear: Ignoring these 3D realities and just "acting as if" is not enough. The 3D reality we live in encompasses our physical world and everyday experiences. For those with challenging backgrounds, the 3D reality is often filled with pain and limitations that are hard to overlook. Healing these deep wounds is essential to align our energy with our true desires and attract positive outcomes. Manifestation for those with this background demands radical self-healing and fierce compassion. It means confronting and transforming past pain, uprooting limiting beliefs, and cultivating a profound sense of safety and trust within us. Rather than learning to ignore the 3D, it's time to face it and heal it.

Acknowledging that manifestation is fundamentally different for those with toxic upbringings is not just empowering—it's revolutionary. By integrating rigorous healing practices with manifestation techniques, and fully embracing our 3D realities, we can shatter our past limitations and unlock our true potential.

I had to get creative and turn metaphysics on its head. Because my mind showed me that when things were good, something was inevitably going to fall apart. That was what my body was conditioned to believe. My secret was that my body had to be retrained, not just my mind. This explained the gaslighting I felt when I looked at the manifestation community. They showed me it was all rainbows and sprinkles when in fact it was very different for me. And it's different for you if you've ever experienced some form of trauma. The secret and the lessons I learned from my father taught me that, yes, I could swim in the stream of life, but for me (and others who looked like me), I was swimming against the current, not with it. Because that's how the stream was designed. This doesn't mean that I can't have what I want. It just means that I must take a different approach to get it, and you might too. Now before you say anything, because I know how some of you like to tussle, take a deep breath and repeat after me: "I am more than what I've been shown, and I can have anything I want."

Choosing Our Path

WHY AM I CHOOSING THIS LIFE? This is the biggest question you'll ask on this journey through the canyon, and quite frankly it might be the hardest. After you get the truth, you might sit in that truth for a little while and work to grasp it. It might get you stuck because the truth hurts at times. It can be painful because truth requires honesty, and so does choice. But this is the pain of creation.

At this point during your journey in the canyon, you might be in limbo. *Should I dwell in the truth for a little longer, or should I get honest with myself and make a choice about what I want?* Honesty is the core of your soul. At times, you are raised to be dishonest with yourself and others around you. You get to a point where you feel so uncomfortable telling the truth that you want to believe the lie. The truth may reveal things about yourself that you feel others will not accept or be able to handle. The truth exposes you to judgment and criticism that you may not be equipped to handle.

So hiding behind that truth becomes a way of life and a badge of honor, and people cannot see the true you.

Dishonesty shows up in your life in many ways. You have conditioned yourself to not tell the truth about little things: not asking for the right salary, not speaking up when people hurt you, and not telling the truth of your desires. You program yourself to downplay things that could possibly bring you joy. Because society has told you that what you want might just be too good to be true, you lie.

Dishonesty manifests itself very subtly. At first, you ignore things that bother you, and then you attempt to convince yourself that what you wanted in the first place is not what you wanted at all. Your dishonesty may not even be your own. It could be something that a parent instilled in you, and you believed their truth instead of your own. Imagine if you lived a life where honesty was the only policy, where there was no room for you to lie to yourself and others around you. Just think about the freedom that holds. Feel that. You would no longer have to hide who you truly are. You could be free. Your soul would thank you for taking that brave step. It would be uncomfortable, but it would be your truth. You wouldn't be able to tolerate anything less from yourself or others.

First, you must ask yourself: *What am I hiding from the world around me?* Once you've identified those things, you must figure out how you plan to rectify those injustices that you've created for yourself. And lastly, you must commit to telling your truth, no matter what, going forward. You must bare it all when you need to or in moments when you want to hide behind old lies. When you are dishonest, you remove the chance for people to get to know the real you. You take the option away from them. That is selfish. Imagine forming a relationship with someone and weeks or months later the "real" them is revealed. You will feel—and probably have felt—betrayed. You question the connection and the truth of what transpired between you and the other person. You then build a wall, and you close yourself up, and that changes your experience with others in the world. Of course, you think, *I wasn't the one who was being dishonest*, but now put the shoe on the other foot and recognize how you might have done that to someone else.

Being honest about what you are choosing in this life is a revolutionary act. When you look in the mirror, you want to know that who you see is who others see as well. You don't want to live a life full of blurred lines. When you start down this road and commit to being honest, you will become mindful of the little lies you tell yourself. This starts with your basic happiness. This begins with your joy. Next, it's crucial to investigate what is important to you. You can't continue to downplay your needs and desires. You have to ask for what you want without fear of people judging you.

Being honest must be a priority. It gives you the opportunity to show up in a world where people are hiding who they really are. You get the chance to be your own person without depending on any external validation. You can stand alone and walk in your truth, feeling the spirits supporting and validating you. Being honest is living in your truth. Dishonesty is hiding behind something that you're not. It's not who you were meant to be. Honesty requires confidence, and dishonesty is insecure.

Take full responsibility for not being honest with yourself. Take full responsibility for allowing yourself to succumb to a standard that never served you in the first place. You can be free, but you first must be willing to let your old self die. You must be willing to lay all your demons down. You must be willing to face your canyon head-on and look yourself in the eyes and tell the truth. The absolute truth. No holding back. No sugarcoating anything to make others or yourself feel safe.

The embodiment of choice connects you to the life you are now choosing after healing parts of yourself, and this teaches you how to trust and be honest with who you are becoming, through metaphysics. To ask the question *Who am I choosing to be?* is to ask *What am I willing to be honest about in my life?* For many years, I hid in this part of the canyon due to my own self-destructive instincts and lack of belief in myself. I was incapable of being honest about what I wanted for my life. For such a long time, I straddled the fence of *Can I have this?* and *Will the world even allow me to have this?*

When my peers were accomplishing societal milestones like getting married and buying homes and climbing the corporate ladder, I knew that I wanted to help people and show them that what they had been birthed into was not all there was, that they could indeed create something different. For goodness' sake, I learned creation from a man who had a BA in accounting but later became a drug dealer. Quite frankly, anything was possible. I just needed to believe that in my body for myself.

Understanding Metaphysics

UNIVERSAL ENERGY DIDN'T DICTATE OUR FATE, but it can be employed to help us along the journey, which is a hell of a lot more empowering than living in a chaotic universe with no shape or form! Universal energy is the gap between the tangible world we see and perceive and the intangible. It's the hidden meaning behind numbers, the bird feathers floating on the breeze while you are walking down the street, or the hummingbird that hovers near your windowsill every day. This energy is a foundational fabric of everything that exists. It's powerful, and it connects us all and sustains everything.

Where there are physical laws and scientific understanding, universal energy occupies the space where spirituality and science intersect. In eastern philosophies, such as Hinduism and Buddhism, this concept is embodied in the notion of prana, or "life force," and is integral to a holistic view of the universe and life. These ideas also parallel the Chinese concept of chi (or qi) in Taoism and traditional Chinese medicine, which describes a vital force that flows through all living entities and is essential for health and vitality.

The western philosophical traditions also had similar ideas. The ancient Greeks conceptualized a form of life energy known as pneuma, an essential spirit of force animating living beings. That idea evolved in the Middle Ages and was reinvented during the Renaissance, as mystical and alchemical ideas were mixed. From a scientific perspective, energy is defined as a measurable property that can be transferred to an object to perform work and can be converted into different forms. Physics recognizes several forms of energy, such as kinetic, potential, thermal, and electromagnetic.

Metaphysics

The scientific perspective on universal energy is rooted in evidence and measurement, which stands in contrast to an abstract spiritual interpretation of universal energy. When we mix in spiritual and metaphysical perspectives, they often focus on the intangible flow of energy in the universe, which can't be quantified through traditional methods.

But recently, we are learning that there is a huge intersection between these spiritual concepts and science when it comes to quantum mechanics and universal energy. Nonetheless, the scientific community generally maintains a distinction between the physically measurable energies studied in physics and the more metaphysical or spiritual concept of a universal energy. This ongoing dialogue between science and spirituality is part of our human quest to understand how it all works together. Drawing from my journey, I recognize the profound significance of universal energy, a concept that transcends the boundaries of conventional understanding.

Through my own experiences and insights, I've come to appreciate that this energy is more than a mere abstract idea; it's a presence that can be felt, sensed, and even harnessed for healing, guidance, and personal growth. It's like an invisible thread connecting everything in the cosmos, a source of wisdom and insight that can be tapped into through intuition and spiritual practice. This energy is not just a philosophical concept but a living, breathing essence that interacts with us in profound and often mysterious ways. From a scientific perspective, universal energy might be seen as elusive, something that eludes empirical measurement and analysis. However, in the realms of spirituality and metaphysics, it's a fundamental truth, a vital force that animates all of existence. I see this as bridging the gap between the seen and the unseen, the physical and the metaphysical.

Doubt in the Canyon

EMBRACING THE CONCEPT OF METAPHYSICS hasn't been without its challenges. Skepticism has been a persistent voice in the back of my head, and likely yours, whispering doubts: *Is this just wishful thinking, a desperate attempt to find meaning in the chaos? Can I really connect to things and people from the other side? Is there even an "other side"?* Scientific explanations often feel more concrete, devoid of the mystical elements that make me feel a little . . . silly as hell.

However, the emotional impact of a belief in metaphysics is undeniable. The moments of peace and guidance, like finding my way out of the woods, are too profound to ignore. The creative surges, seemingly out of nowhere, feel like a gift, a connection to something larger than me. Perhaps the true challenge lies not in denying the unseen, but in finding a way to reconcile it with the world of reason and science. It's a constant dance, this exploration of the seen and unseen, but the journey itself feels deeply meaningful.

I ask you to take a moment and think about a time when you wanted to change your life, and it was hard to believe that anything could be different. But somehow, you trusted the unseen, trusted something bigger than yourself, and your world started to shift. We have all had these moments, these leaps of faith, where logic or reason or friends or family told us we couldn't create or change something, and yet we did. We trusted a future we couldn't yet see, and we made it real.

Your goal through the canyon is not just to understand this universal energy but to help yourself and others connect with it, to use it as a tool for transformation and self-realization. This journey, this exploration of universal energy, is more than a speculative exercise; it's a personal, spiritual quest. It's about peeling back the layers of reality, uncovering the hidden truths that lie beyond the physical world, and tapping into a source of wisdom and power that has been recognized and revered by countless cultures and spiritual traditions throughout history. It's an endeavor that can inspire and challenge you, driving you forward to your mission to enlighten and empower yourself and those around you.

When you lean in to metaphysics, you must keep in mind that your journey is and will be different from that of others who have journeyed in this canyon. Metaphysics offers a multitude of pathways that intertwine your personal and ancestral experiences, which ultimately guide you toward your purpose and destiny.

The journey is not just about learning techniques. It's about unraveling the layers of your existence to reveal the most authentic version of yourself.

When you form rituals and routines that honor your natural connection to source, you can formulate practices that honor your soul. Meditation has always been a foundational practice in metaphysics, but meditation can be more than just quieting the mind and sitting to hear the word of source. You can do this with binaural beats, which is my favorite, or you can get into movement, walking or gardening or being near water. The goal is for you to delve into the inner world of your soul and confront and heal on a personal and ancestral level.

The more you are willing to take a breath and listen to your natural psychic abilities, the more they will become available to you and can guide you toward making choices that serve you better in this life and the next.

Our dreams are also a direct line to our subconscious. In this realm where our deepest truths and hidden fears reside, we can bring forth the choices that we may have trouble making in the psychical world. Your dreams are as powerful and important as breathing.

When you tap into the power of your dreams, you allow yourself to open to the guidance that your soul wants to connect you to. The messages and symbols and patterns in them reflect your journey and bring to light things that may be ignored.

When I have recurring dreams, I take a close look at all the symbolism, from colors to sounds to people to anything that I can recognize that can help in the physical world. My grandmother taught me that dreams are god's way of talking to you without you getting fresh and talking back. It's a one-way communication that allows you to get answers so you can make sound choices. My grandmother got her answers by working with her hands. She had a deep connection to nature and to making things. She spent time outdoors observing the cycles of the sky and weather. She understood that spirit operated in many ways, and she would remind me of that connection (and still does from the afterlife).

You too can develop a relationship with source where you can tap in and birth a new way of feeling through the world. When you are in this part of the canyon, part of you has an idea of what you want and why you are making a choice for your life, but another part of you is fearful of the lack of possibilities because of what you are used to. There will be many times when you will not get the answers you are looking for because you are afraid of the question.

It's time to make a choice that caters to your wildest dream.

I like to say if spirit put it in your heart, it's yours to have. Your only job is to turn your dream into reality. It's your choice. A past life brought you here knowing that there was still more for you to learn, more to challenge you and those around you. Healing old wounds to understand your soul's journey is what this choice is about.

Metaphysics

Choose Which Leg

METAPHYSICS CONNECTS US TO CHOICE BECAUSE it makes us become unwavering in our desires. Choice doesn't tell us to compromise. It asks, *What do you really want and desire?* However, we think that we are supposed to take less than what we've asked for, and that is not true. When we look at the word *choice*, it's the act of selecting or making decisions when faced with possibilities. Choice says to us that we have autonomy and freedom to decide what we want based on our preferences, needs, values, and desires. We are faced with choices every day, from what we want to eat for breakfast to more consequential decisions. Sometimes we are even faced with decisions that can propel our life in one direction or another.

When I was growing up in New York City and getting ready to go to high school, I was given a choice to apply to specific schools to concentrate on a vocation. I wanted to be an architect. About two years prior, I had been living in Atlanta, and one of my classes in the sixth grade was architecture. Our teacher was a Black man who was part of the national organization of minority architects, and he was always impressed with the way I completed my assignments. I was efficient and did them fast while following instructions to a T.

One day, as he was handing me back an assignment, he said, "You're good at this. You should think about making this a career." I felt happy that someone saw something special in me. I rarely heard words of encouragement, just words that shut down my creativity. So when my mother and I moved back to Queens when I was thirteen years old, I knew that I wanted to be an architect, but unfortunately when I got to high school, I didn't do well in an environment with a six to one ratio of boys to girls. The overwhelming number of male interests I received created constant distractions, such as multiple young men calling my house. At one point I had four different boys whose names all started with the letter D calling my house. This made it difficult to focus and thrive academically in that setting.

All the attention I paid to the young men at school sparked my interest in fashion. I decided to move in a different direction. I was failing most of my classes because I was more concerned with boys than with my books. But that changed fast when my mom switched me out of that school. I got a fresh start somewhere else where I was able to thrive. This is how choices can affect us. These choices can be good, or they can be not so favorable. We make important choices every day; we decide between two different job offers, select a vacation destination, and choose people to hang out with, date, and marry.

When it comes to metaphysics and the nature of your soul, you might ask, *Do I really have a choice?* And you might argue, *What about free will?* There is an old-school psychic I know of who says, "Free will is god/source/spirit telling you to lift your leg, and you choose which leg to lift."

That explanation made it clear that the choices we are given and faced with are always divine and they are intended to keep us on the path that our soul came here to journey. You may think you have fallen behind or are on the wrong path because there are things that you are experiencing that leave you unsure about your next steps, but you are being guided, whether you like it or not.

Metaphysics and choice go hand in hand because you are making choices that align with your true self and what you value. The metaphysical exploration of your identity leads to a deeper understanding of how and why you make the choices you do. Our perception of what we see in our present can dictate the choices we make, and this can be very skewed when you are in the canyon because you are looking at your choices based on what you currently know. The possibilities may not yet be available in the mind that you are currently using.

I use metaphysics to embody choice in listening to the nudges that I get. It allows me to work with the universal energy and trust that what's for me will be in alignment with what I've been shown from spirit, via dreams or downloads. It helps me create rituals that help me surrender to my personal manifestation process, showing me how things work. I know that I have control over my life, but I also know there is a time for everything.

Your Magical Motherfucking Download

There are several ways to tap into your natural creation process by using the elements of fire, air, water, and earth in order to create the life you desire and see where your soul is guiding you. I believe that this level of creation is based on the divine masculine and divine feminine. Everyone, no matter the gender, has both divine masculine and divine feminine within them, and for the purposes of creation and choice, you need both to answer the question What do I truly want to create in this life?

The divine masculine can act and assert itself and has a clear direction in life. It's about rational thinking and structure when approaching life's challenges. It is disciplined and focused while using determination to pursue goals.

The divine feminine is about using an innate sense of knowing and creativity to make something out of thin air. Emotional intelligence leads the way to deeply empathize with the world around you. The divine feminine is adaptable, flows with life's rhythms, and is open to receiving.

The masculine and feminine are represented within you no matter your gender, and both are needed for creation. You can create the life you desire by tapping into your sun and moon astrological placements.

The sun is associated with the masculine because it represents the basic version of your identity, ego, and sense of self. It's the version of you that people remember. It's your conscious and active mind, how your mind rationally thinks. The sun's energy is about clarity and the lens you use as you pursue your truth. It's your life force, how you lead, and the path you are meant to follow to fulfill your potential.

The moon is associated with the feminine because it represents your emotions and moods and how you intuitively respond to the world. It's how you care for yourself and how you care for others. It symbolizes your capacity to adapt to changing circumstances. It's your inner world when no one is around. It's where you process and internalize your choices and experiences and your environment.

When you are in the canyon, you can use the elements to help guide you toward why you are choosing this life. You get to decide how you want to lead. Remember, masculine and feminine are not gender-specific, so if you are choosing to lead your choice of creation through the masculine energy, you will focus on your sun sign first, then your moon. If you are choosing to lead your choice of creation through the feminine energy, you will focus on your moon sign first, then your sun.

If your sun or moon is in the fire element—which I call the catalyst of transformation and passion—your purpose in this part of the canyon is to change and transform raw energy into your deepest passions. It's about using this power to transform your life and your surroundings. Fire represents not just a physical energy but the inner passion of your spirit. It's the part of you that seeks a challenge and seeks growth. Your goal is to engage in rituals where you can visualize burning away the old version of you and calling in the new version of you. Writing can act as a metaphorical fire, helping you channel and transform your thoughts and emotions. Use the energy of fire to stop procrastinating and initiate new projects. When you aren't motivated or when you face resistance, use fire to ignite your enthusiasm and determination.

If your sun or moon is in the air element—which I call the power of thoughts and communication—your purpose in this part of the canyon is to spark new ideas. Air governs the realm of thoughts and ways to communicate your ideas in the world. It represents mental clarity and the power of intention, which is the invisible force that connects all things. Use this energy to give form to thoughts and ideas. Your qualities are best applied with clear thinking, alert decision-making, and innovative solutions.

If your sun or moon is in the water element—which I call emotions, intuition, and the flow of life—your purpose in this part of the canyon is to tap into your emotional response and the depth of your feelings, to let your psychic energies flow. Water represents a fluid and adaptable energy that can wield power by tapping into all the emotions. Use this energy to understand and manage your emotions both personally and universally.

If your sun or moon is in the earth element, which I call grounding, materialization, and stability, your purpose in this part of the canyon is to focus on the tangible, material aspects of life and your physical body in terms of your environment and your foundation. Earth represents everything about grounding your dreams and being in a stable environment. Use this energy when you are seeking to manifest goals, especially those related to physical well-being, career, and home. When you feel uncertain, draw in the earth's energy to remain centered and balanced.

Harnessing the Energies

IN OUR JOURNEY OF SELF-HEALING AND discovery through the canyon, the elemental forces of air, fire, water, and earth serve as more than mere symbols; they are vital confidants that guide us through our inner worlds as we venture to heal and integrate the shadow parts of ourselves. Each element, deeply rooted in various spiritual, astrological, and natural systems, offers unique energies and lessons, allowing us to connect more profoundly with the universe and the deepest parts of our being.

The element of air symbolizes intellect, communication, and clarity. It's the breath of life, the unseen wind that whispers wisdom and truth. In our daily lives, we can invoke the essence of air to bring clarity to our thoughts, to lift the veil that shrouds our deeper understanding. This is especially crucial in the canyon when confronting those concealed, often neglected aspects of our psyches. Through practices like deep and intentional breathing, meditation, and engaging conversations, we can harness the power of air. This element helps us articulate and navigate through the complex entanglement of emotions and thoughts that dwell in the canyon, enabling us to see with greater clarity and understanding.

Fire, with its raw energy and transformative power, symbolizes passion, courage, and regeneration. It is both the spark that ignites the flames of change and the warmth that fosters growth and resilience. In the canyon, fire emboldens us to confront our deepest fears and to embrace our inner strengths. It's about igniting the internal flame to burn away old beliefs, fears, and habits, making room for new growth and transformation. Simple yet profound practices like illuminating our space with candles, basking in the warmth of the sun, engaging in physical activities, or pursuing creative endeavors like painting or writing can be powerful methods to channel the transformative energy of fire into our daily lives. This element teaches us the art of rebirth—how to rise from the ashes of our old selves, renewed and empowered.

The element of water, fluid and ever-changing, represents emotion, intuition, and the subconscious. It is the deep, nurturing force that teaches us about the depth of our feelings and the power of adaptation. Engaging with the element of water means diving into the deepest parts of our emotional selves, uncovering hidden wounds, and gently healing them. This can be beautifully symbolized and practiced through rituals like taking cleansing baths or simply being near bodies of water. Water teaches us the importance of emotional flow, of acknowledging and releasing emotions to prevent stagnation, thereby promoting profound emotional healing and intuition.

The element of earth, the ultimate symbol of stability, fertility, and grounding, shows us our connection to the physical world. In our journey through the canyon, earth reminds us of the importance of being grounded and present. It's about connecting to the physical senses, nourishing the body, and finding stability and safety within ourselves. Practices such as gardening, mindful eating, engaging in nature walks, and yoga allow us to connect with the earth element. These activities help us stay rooted and balanced, providing a strong foundation as we explore the more ethereal aspects of our being.

Combining these elements—air, fire, water, and earth—into our daily routines and healing practices offers an approach to understanding and nurturing our whole selves. They encourage us to embrace every facet of our existence, including the canyon, and to harness these energies as allies in our journey toward self-discovery, healing, and ultimately transformation.

As you incorporate these elements into your life, let them be a reminder of your deep connection to the universe, your inner strength, and your ability to evolve and thrive through every phase of your life's journey.

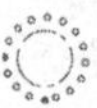

METAPHYSICS SHOWS US HOW TO get out of a bad job or a bad relationship, just as it can guide us to the right job or the right partner. But even more than that, metaphysics allows us to look at ourselves in the mirror and say, "I've got your back, and we can get the life we want."

In the canyon, we find the repressed emotions, traumas, and aspects of our personality that we've disowned due to fear, shame, or societal pressure. It's in the depths of the canyon that metaphysics plays its most crucial role. Through practices like deep meditation, energy work, and astrology, we start a dialogue with these hidden parts. This is not just self-reflection; it's a profound journey of reintegration and understanding.

As we embrace our canyons, we start to see the world and ourselves differently. Our intuition sharpens as a natural consequence of becoming more aligned with our inner truth. This heightened intuition is our psychic ability coming to the forefront. It's a reminder that within each of us lies a vast, untapped potential to connect with something greater than ourselves: the universal consciousness. It's a reminder that our souls choose these moments to evolve into the wholeness of our truest selves.

This journey, however, is not just about developing psychic abilities. It's about healing all the parts of ourselves so that our most authentic selves shine at their brightest. As we heal, we shed layers of false beliefs and imposed identities. We begin to manifest our reality from a place of authenticity. Our thoughts, now more aligned with our true selves, have a profound impact on the reality we create.

Metaphysics

Metaphysics teaches us that our outer world reflects our inner state. If your inner state is riddled with the baggage of your conditioning, it can be hard to reflect the beauty that you were meant to experience in this lifetime. By working through your shadow, you bring light to the darkness within, and this light begins to reflect on every aspect of your life. Your relationships, career, and personal well-being start to resonate with a newfound inner harmony.

This transformation is not always easy. It requires courage, honesty, tenacity, and persistence. But the rewards are boundless. You become a conduit of truth, not just for yourself but for others. Your psychic abilities, now honed and refined, allow you to guide, heal, and inspire those around you. In essence, metaphysics isn't just changing your life; it's redefining it. By healing in the canyon, you're not just finding your true self; you're unlocking your highest potential, both psychic and spiritual. It's a journey of becoming the most enlightened, empowered, and authentic version of yourself, and in doing so, you become a super bright beam in a world that so desperately needs it.

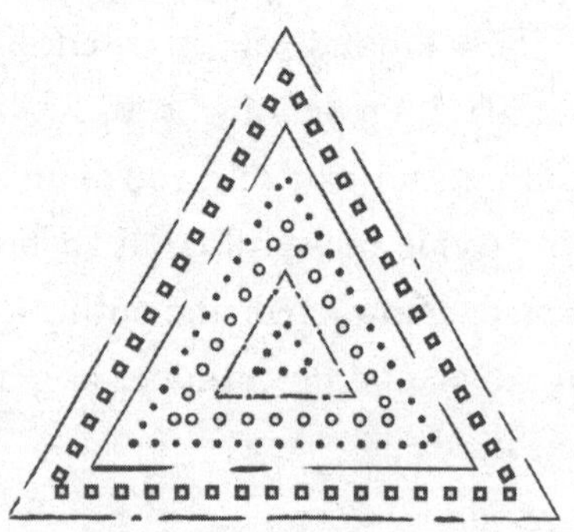

How Do I Want to Change My World and the World Around Me?

7

HUMAN DESIGN FOR LIBERATION

The Embodiment of Change

IMAGINE YOU'RE WALKING TOWARD what you believe is the right path, but something feels off. It feels like something is missing. Every step is deliberate, and it feels like you are headed in the right direction, and yet, you are still strangely lost. College degree? Check. Marketable major? Secured. Decent job on the horizon? Practically guaranteed. Yet a nagging feeling sits in your gut, throwing you off your normal rhythm. It's like there's an invisible resistance pulling you back, a subtle current urging you in a different direction. You push on, putting a smile on your face, trying to drown out the unease. Then you discover a system that rocks your world, making you question everything about your life. And yet, for the first time, everything makes sense.

That's what human design did for me.

I had just moved to the DMV (DC, Maryland, and Virginia area) after having left the New York / New Jersey area where I had lived my entire life, with the exception of a short stint in Atlanta when my parents parted ways. I left New York to start a new life, and just as I was getting started, that life felt like it was crashing down all around me. In New York, I was in acting school and taking classes at NYU SPS (New York University School of Professional Studies), learning film and TV production. I left it all because I fell in love. And I thought that was the path I was supposed to take, but I quickly realized that dropping everything for a relationship wasn't my true path.

I got a job at a metal machinery supplier in the sales department. I started missing my creative endeavors. My partner at the time was a Capricorn, and he had no clue what it meant to "follow your dreams"; he was very practical and critical. In his eyes, the corporate path was the only road to success.

I knew that wasn't true, but I let my fear convince me otherwise. Then I did what I always do, and asked spirit for a sign, and that sign came in a layoff. Though I liked the company, I saw the job loss as a sign to pursue my passion, which at the time was photography. I'm a creative person, and I've always found myself trying new things. From a young age, I was taught that an idle mind is the devil's playground. Pursuing my creative endeavors has given me the opportunity to expand, even in the smallest ways. I started to intern at a commercial photographer's studio, which helped me launch my photography career. I went on to do weddings, portraits, short films, and much more.

One day during my internship, I was talking to the makeup artist, and she was a heavy yogi. We would talk after each photo shoot, and one day she said there is this thing called human design, referring to herself as "a manifestor." I had no idea what she was talking about, but she explained that there were five human design aura types. I listened in awe because I'd never heard of this "human design" thing.

Growing up, I always felt different. As bell hooks says, I was cared for, but not loved and nurtured in the way I needed to be, in the way all children need to be. From a very young age, my mother would at times call me selfish, lazy, and a bitch; I felt like there was something wrong with me. As I grew older, I turned to my psychic gifts and used metaphysical modalities to create new ideas and new thoughts to help me identify and believe in my goals, dreams, and desires. These modalities helped me survive.

When my friend at work told me that she was a manifestor, I figured I was one as well. I manifest things, so of course I would be a manifestor. She told me what website to go to and who to get a reading from. To my surprise, I discovered my human design type: projector. I thought to myself, *This can't be true*. I read that projectors are here to wait to be invited, and I said, "I don't wait for anything. Who the fuck does that?"

I was beyond pissed. I actually cried. What was I supposed to do, just sit around and wait for my life to magically unfold? This system went against everything I had been told as a Black woman: I have to be the best, do the most, and excel no matter what. No excuses. Was that really working for me? Yes and no.

As I began to think about it, my body could never truly keep up

with the pace of everyone else. I had to do things in my own time. *Maybe this projector thing wasn't wrong*, I thought. The woman who did my first reading said, "Invitations are big, especially when it comes to things that will pivot or change the direction of your life."

As I discovered, I come from a family of generators—both my parents and my extended family. I had been pushing myself my whole life, but maybe that was what had been wrong. What if I stopped pushing? The only thing was, the more I learned about human design, the more I realized that there weren't too many people doing it who looked like me. I realized that if I wanted to adopt this modality, I needed to teach it not through the lens of other people's cultures but through my own. Human design is a system that combines principles of astrology, the *I Ching*, kabbalah, and the chakra system to provide a comprehensive blueprint of an individual's unique nature. Created by Ra Uru Hu in 1987, it offers insights into our strengths, challenges, and purpose by mapping out our energy centers and how they interact. By understanding your human design, you can align more closely with your true self and navigate life with greater clarity and ease.

I studied, took classes, and read charts, but I started seeing human design very differently because of the trauma I was working through. And things weren't adding up. First and foremost, I am a Black woman living in a world where people who look like me aren't praised. As the old Black proverb goes, "I have to work twice as hard to get half of what others get," which has always rung true. Additionally, there are natural privileges I haven't been afforded when it comes to career, love, and success. Things have always just looked different for me.

Everyone I found online or on YouTube was loving and lighting the hell out of me and using phrases like "Ra said this" and "Ra said that," and I was like, *Ra doesn't even look like me so what the hell does he know?*

I was right. Ra didn't know my experience; that's why I had to make the system he invented, human design, my own.

So when I started using this system in my work and helping others use the system, my perspective came from a place of being trauma-informed. I knew that love and light were great, but trauma and pain were also real. Though I know there are some who see human design as a cult, I see it as an experiment. And if you learn how to use it to your advantage, it can be an experiment that works. But first you must heal other parts of yourself to truly understand what it is trying to teach you.

For me, human design means that I get my own instruction manual that says if I use this as a guideline to align with everything that is meant for me, then I don't have to force anything. I get to exist in a world that responds to me and shows me not just who I was always meant to be but who I have always been.

A Brief Note About Human Design

I WANT TO PAINT A PICTURE for you. Let's say you devour a memoir, a raw and captivating story that feels like it crawled into your soul and laid your struggles bare. Then, boom! Literary scandal erupts. It turns out that the author, the one who made you feel so seen, fabricated large chunks of the story, à la James Frey's *A Million Little Pieces*. Betrayal stings, leaving you wondering how something so seemingly true but built on lies could have a real impact on your journey.

After reading James Frey's book, being amazed by his writing and story (and absolutely loving the cover design), and watching Oprah Winfrey praise him on her show, I was shocked that the story wasn't completely factual.

This is the headspace many find themselves in with human design. This system, with its birth chart blueprints and energetic personality breakdowns, feels like a revelation. It explains your anxieties, your creative bursts, and the way you interact with the world—a social butterfly or a lone wolf, depending on your "type."

But then you stumble upon the not-so-flattering details about the system's creator, Alan Robert Krakower, also known as Ra Uru Hu. Accusations of racism and classism and a focus on financial gain later in his career cast a shadow on the entire practice, and it's enough to make you want to slam the book shut and walk away from the whole self-discovery thing.

Here's the thing: Just because an author embellished their story doesn't negate the profound impact that story might have on your journey. Human design, like most powerful tools, has a complex past. Its roots delve into ancient wisdom traditions, a tapestry woven from diverse cultures and lineages stretching back millennia. Think of it like a groundbreaking medical treatment—its discovery might be attributed to a controversial figure, but its ability to heal remains undeniable. The embodiment of change is a core principle of human design that connects you to how you impact the world and teaches you how to use your unique energetic blueprint to create your own personal legacy. It's about taking the wisdom of this ancient system and remixing it for your modern life.

We're not worshipping the messenger; we're focusing on the message itself. Even though human design was "downloaded" by a man with a troubled past, the system itself draws from a rich ancestral lineage. I'm not here to erase the truth about human design's origin story, but I also won't let it overshadow the transformative potential it offers. I'll acknowledge the "million little lies" surrounding its creation but celebrate the "billion year wisdom" at its core.

A Little Background on Human Design

HUMAN DESIGN ISN'T A PERSONALITY TEST. It's a deep dive into the user manual you were never given—for yourself!

In 1987, Krakower left his family in Canada and went on a spiritual journey to Ibiza, Spain, for eight days. He encountered a voice, something of a mystical download, that helped him craft an intricate framework called human design.

Human design is a captivating blend of ancient wisdom from various cultures with modern scientific concepts. Human design isn't just another horoscope with a fancy name, even though it utilizes your birth date and time to generate your chart; it delves far deeper than your sun sign. It meticulously examines the precise alignment of the planets at your exact moment of arrival into the realm. This unique snapshot holds the key to your energy, your decision-making, and the way you interact with the world around you.

It's a vibrant tapestry woven with threads of astrology, the *I Ching*, kabbalah, and the Hindu chakra system. These age-old traditions provide the foundation for understanding our energetic makeup. Human design also reaches into the realm of quantum mechanics and genetics, suggesting a fascinating connection between the universe's building blocks and our own bioelectric nature. It's a complex system with several key components, each with roots in ancient wisdom traditions. Here's a glimpse into some of the major parts:

- **The *I Ching*:** Human design's foundation rests on the ancient wisdom of the *I Ching*, a Chinese divination text with a history stretching back over three thousand years. This profound system isn't just about predicting the future; it's a map for understanding the energetic landscape of life. The *I Ching* explores the concept of "chi," the vital life force that flows through all living things. Imagine it as an invisible river coursing through your body and the world around you, influencing everything from your moods to the ebb and flow of life itself. Human design utilizes the *I Ching*'s framework to map your individual chi flow, helping you understand how you interact with this energetic current.
- **The chakra system:** Human design incorporates the concept of chakras, a cornerstone of Hindu and tantric traditions. These aren't just physical locations in the body, but rather swirling vortexes of energy that connect our physical, emotional, and spiritual selves. Each chakra has a specific function and influence on our well-being. By understanding our unique chakra system through the lens of human design, we can learn to cultivate a harmonious flow of energy within ourselves, leading to greater physical, emotional, and spiritual balance.
- **Kabbalah:** Human design draws upon the depths of kabbalah, a mystical tradition within Judaism that scholars have explored for centuries. From this rich wellspring comes the concept of archetypes: universal patterns of energy that resonate within our personalities and life experiences. These archetypes, like the warrior or the healer, can offer insights into our strengths and challenges and the roles we naturally play in the world. Kabbalah

also contributes the idea of life purpose, guiding us toward understanding the unique contribution we are meant to make while we're here. Human design helps us identify our archetype and life purpose, empowering us to live a more authentic and fulfilling journey.

- **Western astrology:** The vast tapestry of human design wouldn't be complete without acknowledging the influence of the cosmos. Human design integrates the wisdom of Western astrology, recognizing the significance of planetary placements on our birth charts. These placements aren't just about sun signs, but rather a complex interplay of celestial energies that shape our unique energetic blueprint. Human design goes beyond simply saying you're a Leo or a Scorpio. It interprets the specific dance of planets within your birth chart, revealing how these cosmic forces influence your energy, personality, and life path.

These are just a few of the threads woven into the tapestry of human design.

This is your invitation to embark on an exploration with open eyes. We'll delve into the fascinating world of human design, exploring the embodiment of change and how it connects you to your purpose and the legacy you want to leave behind. We'll dissect the system, not to idolize its creator but to unlock its power for personal growth and positive change in the world.

Even flawed systems can hold profound wisdom. As a mentor, teacher, and consultant who guides others, my past is far from perfect. However, my past doesn't erase the valuable lessons that I can teach and guide others through. With human design, you'll learn to harness this wisdom, navigate its complexities, and ultimately use it to create a life that's authentically you—a legacy built on your own truth, not someone else's.

A Portrait of Liberation

HUMAN DESIGN IS A POTENT BLEND of ancient wisdom and modern science that reveals the way that you uniquely interact with the world and the power you hold to create positive change within your life and the lives of those around you.

Human design is not just a personality test. It uses your birthplace, birth time, and birth date to unlock a deep wellspring of energy that not only fuels your purpose but guides you toward your path to personal liberation. It is also the liberation that you use as fuel in the world around you. Human design paints your energetic portrait with a concept called aura types. Think of your aura as an energetic field that surrounds you and also is within you. It influences how you interact with the world and how the world interacts with and responds to you.

There are five distinct aura types, each with its own rhythm and flow: you have generators, manifesting generators, projectors, manifestors, and reflectors. Every aura type moves in the world a certain way, and the world responds to each in a certain way. When we look at human design from a liberation standpoint, we are gauging how our energetic blueprints can free us from societal pressures and from societal expectations.

Even though human design was created at the height of capitalism and forged a path to categorize people in a classist way (as workers, builders, or leaders), it often failed to recognize the inherent socioeconomic differences between those roles. This oversight can lead to a narrow interpretation of one's potential and capabilities that ignores the broader context of social and economic factors that influence an individual's opportunities and life path.

It's important to approach human design with a critical eye, understanding that while it offers valuable insights into our innate traits and tendencies, it must be balanced with an awareness of the external circumstances that shape our experiences. By doing so, we can use human design as a tool for empowerment rather than limitation, fostering a more inclusive and equitable understanding of human potential.

Human design gives you the opportunity to ask yourself, *How do I want to change my world and the world around me?* or *How do I want to respond to the world, and how do I want the world to respond to me?*

Have you ever noticed how some people seem to effortlessly command attention, while others thrive by responding to their environment? This captivating dance between inner energy and the outside world is a core principle in human design. It all boils down to your aura type, a unique blueprint that defines how you interact with the world and tap into your life force. Now is the perfect time to go and find your human design type and get the lay of the land for your natural energies.

Imagine yourself basking in the sunshine, your energy field radiating outward like a luminous sphere, constantly pulsing with a specific kind of energy. That, my friend, is your aura, and in human design, it holds the key to unlocking your life's rhythm. Now, auras aren't one-size-fits-all. There are actually five distinct types, each with its own unique way of interacting with the world. They're like the essential instruments in a killer band—all vital, but each bringing a special flavor to the song of life. The bass player lays down the foundation, the drums keep the beat pumping, the guitar riffs ignite the melody, the keyboard weaves intricate harmonies, and the vocals deliver the soul-stirring message.

Generators

Generators are the energizers of the aura types. Imagine an engine that thrives on responding to life. Generators are fueled by a deep guttural knowing or the sacral response that tells you when to step in and act. The question for generators isn't *Should I do this?* but rather *Does this resonate with my inner hum, my inner feeling, my inner nature?*

Generators are natural cocreators. They partner with the right people, projects, or situations that ignite their internal yes, and when they do that, you can watch and see their energy spark a positive change. Many people think that generators and manifesting generators are very similar, but I strongly disagree. In my view, generators are more akin to projectors than to manifesting generators. While generators are often categorized in the same family as manifesting generators, I see them as more like cousins rather than siblings. The distinctions between these types are significant and shouldn't be overlooked.

Manifesting Generators

Manifesting generators are a force of nature with a dash of diplomacy. Manifesting generators possess a potent blend of unstoppable drive and strategic charm. I like to say that manifesting generators are powerhouses but with permission; they need to inform the world of their intentions before diving in. They work best when they say to people, "Heads up! I'm about to do something great in the world." This simple act of informing not only respects the energies of those around them but also helps them tap into their own power source. When manifesting generators announce their initiatives, they ignite collaboration and witness the ripple effect of their actions. They can be a wave of inspiration to others around them.

Projectors

Projectors are guides who are here on this earth to see the potential in others. They are here to guide and direct other people's energies. Projectors possess a captivating aura that draws out the best in everyone around them, but the key is that they need an invitation to share their wisdom and guidance. Projectors are not here to force anything. They are here to trust that the right opportunities will arise for them and illuminate a path for themselves and others. Projectors are here to become a magnetic guide who empowers others to step into their most powerful selves, to step into their brilliance.

When projectors recognize those who resonate with their energy, they are able to offer insights with clarity, compassion, and kindness. The projector energy says, "I see you."

Manifestors

Manifestors are very bold initiators; they operate on a completely different frequency. They are not here to ask for permission. Manifestors don't need permission. They are here to inform others about their actions after they've taken them or to inform others of what is going to happen next. This can be disruptive to those around them, but it is their natural way of igniting change. Manifestors are trailblazers who carve out new paths. When they clearly communicate their intentions, they watch how their decisive actions inspire everyone around them to take the lead in their own lives. Manifestors have a lot of power because they need courage within themselves to move forward with their ideas, with their passions, with their dreams, and with their way of being in order to move the collective around them.

Reflectors

Reflectors are wisdom mirrors. They are the most sensitive yet nuanced aura type. They absorb and reflect the energy of everyone around them. They are always evolving, depending on their environment. They have a very chameleonic nature, which for them can feel very overwhelming at times, but it is their superpower. Reflectors embrace their role as a living mirror; they are here to reflect the truth back into any environment that they are in. They surround themselves with positive, growth-oriented people as they watch their own path of positive change unfold; and when it unfolds, it will unfold organically.

Our energetic blueprint is undeniably shaped by our experiences, including past traumas. These experiences leave behind self-parts, fragmented aspects of ourselves, and they cause us to hold on to pain and limiting beliefs. Human design combined with trauma healing modalities can be a powerful tool for integrating these parts in stepping into your full potential.

When you think about human design, know that it isn't just a static image. It's a pulsating energetic flow through nine distinct centers. Gates and channels and planets comprise a blueprint that influences how you experience that energy. I want you to imagine your chart as a map of your energetic landscape. When you recognize centers that may be blocked or undefined due to trauma, you can begin to work on healing and integrating. This might involve practices of canyon work, inner child work, or somatic therapies. As you heal the past, your energetic flow becomes smoother, allowing you to embody your design fully.

The main mechanics of human design, especially what you'll need as you work through the canyon, really come down to your aura type, your strategy, and your authority. This helps you know the truth about how you can change your world and the world around you.

This is the next step in trusting yourself. This is the truth in knowing what's right for you will be for you, based on your strategy and authority. Human design helps you do things differently and accept your own personal destiny to create an impactful life on a personal level. It influences you across all areas of life.

Your Magical Motherfucking Download

Your human design chart or body graph is your blueprint, and it has a signature that you carry out throughout your life.

Each of the five different human design aura types has a different signature: generators' and manifesting generators' signature is satisfaction, projectors' is success, manifestors' is peace, and reflectors' is surprise. Once you identify your aura, your signature, and the other key elements of your chart, you will better understand how to use human design to change your outer world. Human design offers a simple framework for understanding yourself and interacting with the world more authentically.

Here are some embodied practices for change tailored to each aura type, helping you live in your signature and create a more fulfilling life.

Embodied Practices for Generators

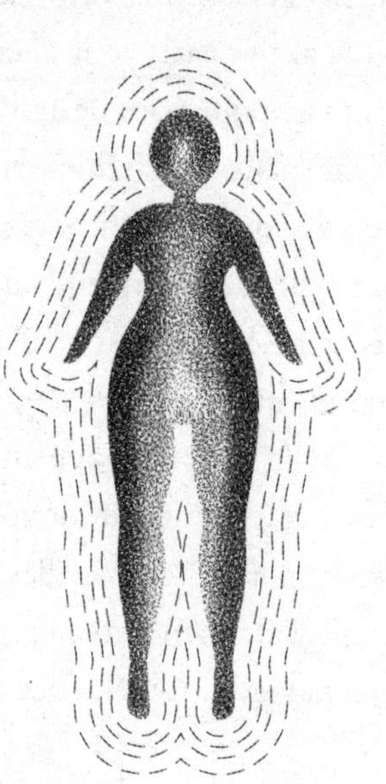

Generators' signature is satisfaction. The key to generators' satisfaction lies in responding to what lights them up. If you are a generator, an embodied practice for you to take on is movement. Move your body. Find activities that ignite your sacral response, whether it's dancing, martial arts, sports, or anything that gets your energy flowing. The goal is to notice an internal *umph* of satisfaction as you engage in these activities. This is your inner compass guiding you toward fulfilling experiences. When you are living your signature, instead of forcing action you are waiting for the *umph* before taking the next step.

Forcing action means trying to make things happen out of alignment with your natural flow and timing. It involves pushing yourself to do things because you think you should, rather than because it feels right or the timing is appropriate. This often leads to frustration and burnout. Instead, when you wait for the *umph*, that internal signal or feeling of readiness, you move forward with more ease and authenticity, aligned with your authentic self and the right timing. You must say no to opportunities that don't resonate, and trust your sacral wisdom to guide you toward fulfilling projects and relationships.

A few ways to do this are writing down your gut feelings and tracking the energy behind them. What feels like a resounding *yes* to you? What feels like a draining *no*? When you explore practices like yoga or dance to reconnect with the physical sensations and your intuition in your body, you heal past experiences of invalidation. Make sure you are constantly checking in with your inner child to allow them to shine as their most authentic self.

Embodied Practices for Manifesting Generators

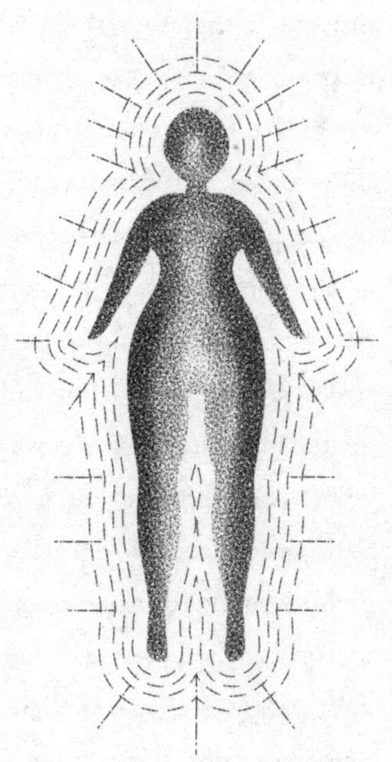

For manifesting generators, similar to generators, their signature is satisfaction. Manifesting generators thrive on responding to what feels good, but they also benefit from informing others of their desires. The embodied practice for a manifesting generator is vocal expression.

Practice expressing your desires verbally. This could be through affirmations, role-playing with a friend, or journaling your desires. The goal is to notice how your body responds: Do you feel a sense of clarity or a settling feeling that indicates alignment? As a manifesting generator, your voice is your lifeline. When you speak, imagine your words vibrating through the ethers of the universe. Living your signature means listening for that sacral *umph* of satisfaction, then informing others of your intentions before acting. Whether you're seeking permission or simply announcing your plans, this clear communication attracts opportunities that resonate with your desires.

Manifesting generators also need to explore practices where they can verbalize their needs and desires. They need to heal their inner child by validating their voice, whether that's through singing, chanting, talking to others, or doing activities where they can connect their voice to their body.

Embodied Practices for Projectors

Projectors' signature is success. This one is tricky because success means different things to different people. Projectors thrive on being recognized for their unique gifts. However, success doesn't always come from self-promotion. Sometimes success arises from being really good at just existing and then being invited into situations or environments where you can share your expertise and experiences. Projectors are here to embody energetic awareness.

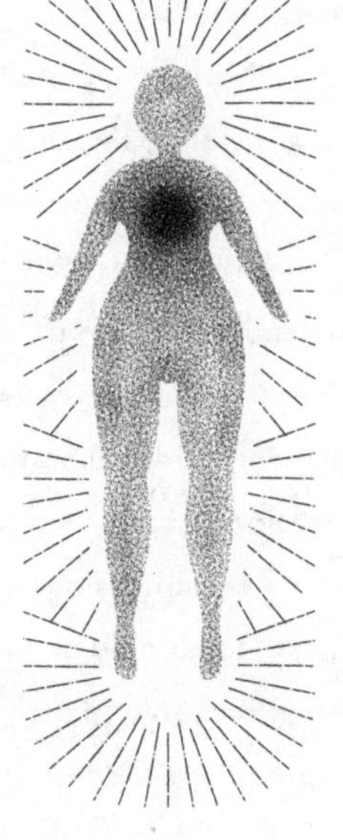

Notice when you feel a sense of anticipation or excitement around a person or opportunity. This is your inner compass guiding you toward invitations for success. It is key for you, as a projector, to understand what and who makes you feel good. When you are living in your signature, you are developing skills and expertise in areas that resonate with you and make you feel whole. You must cultivate patience and trust that the right invitations will come when you are energetically aligned with the situation. When invited to share your insights, do so with confidence. Know your value. As you journey through the canyon, your goal is to set boundaries. Practice saying no to requests that drain your energy. Throughout life you are going to have to discern invitations. You are going to have to learn to differentiate between exploring opportunities to succeed and just doing things for the sake of people-pleasing. As you develop self-worth and confidence in your unique gifts you will not need validation.

Anytime you find yourself needing external validation, you are not aligned. Seeking approval from others can pull you away from your true self and create a disconnect from your inner guidance. Instead, reorient by focusing on opportunities that spark excitement you can feel in your body. This embodied excitement is a signal that you are on the right path and aligned with your authentic self.

Embodied Practices for Manifestors

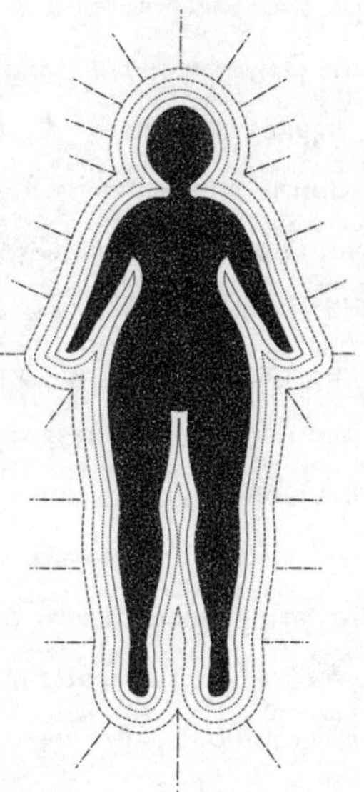

Manifestors' signature is peace. Manifestors find peace by informing others of their intentions and acting without waiting for permission. To embody peace as a manifestor, you must develop assertive communication. Practice clear and assertive (not aggressive) communication. It's about stating your needs and desires and boundaries with confidence. Pay attention to your body: A sense of calm and ease indicates alignment; living your signature means trusting your gut instinct. When you feel called to act, inform others of your intention without seeking permission, then follow through. Respect the boundaries of others, but remain true to your own by any means necessary. Stay true to the course.

As a manifestor, you need to develop emotional intelligence while you're in the canyon. You need to develop empathy and learn to read the emotional landscape of others. This is not to put other people first, but rather to understand how people might respond to your initiations. When you get comfortable explaining your "why," you can act. Work on being understood so you can express your authority with confidence.

Embodied Practices for Reflectors

The reflectors' signature is surprise. In a way, reflectors don't have a predefined signature because they thrive on experiencing life's full spectrum. Reflecting the energies of those around them is just as important as the air that they breathe.

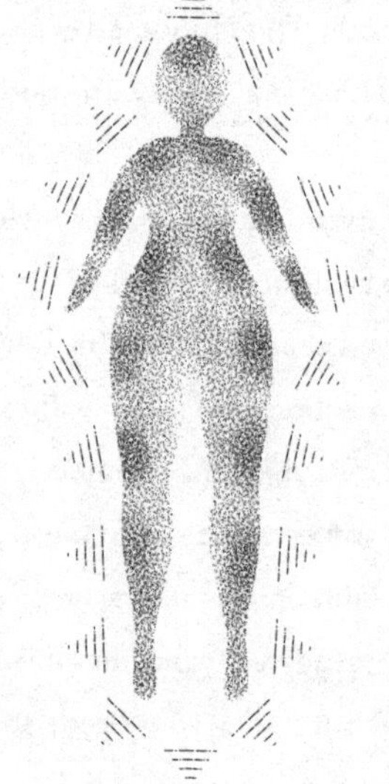

If you are a reflector, an embodied practice that you need to adapt while in the canyon is sensory exploration. Learn to engage your senses fully. Notice the sights, sounds, smells, tastes, and textures around you. Spend time in environments that are different from what you're used to. Try new foods. Surround yourself with diverse people. This openness allows you to absorb the world and find your unique place in it. To live your signature, it is important for you to avoid making quick decisions; you are here to spend time with different people and in different environments, allowing yourself to reflect and absorb their energy.

You must trust that clarity and direction will emerge organically as you experience life unfolding. It is important for you to learn how to curate your environment, spending time with supportive people and in nurturing spaces that uplift your energy. You must learn how to differentiate your own energy from the energies that you are picking up from other people. Solitude and meditation can help with that. Self-care rituals are important prioritizing activities that nourish your mind, body, and soul. Expressing and journaling about your needs are great ways to confidently and clearly communicate your needs when someone asks about them in person or in any social interaction.

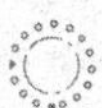

Human design allows you to embrace the different energies that you may interact with—such as frustration, anger, or insecurity—and provides help if you find yourself mirroring past experiences. Human design will allow you to reframe these challenges as opportunities for learning and transformation. For example, a generator who thrives on action might find a projectors' waiting to be recognized frustrating. Human design can help them understand that this frustration might stem from childhood experiences of invalidation. By recognizing these triggers, the generator can communicate their needs more effectively, and the projector can learn to express their value more openly. This fosters a more collaborative and supportive dynamic.

Human design helps you embrace those triggers to transformation but also encourages us to move beyond a one-size-fits-all approach to the world. If we can appreciate the unique energetic makeup of each person, we can cultivate more respectful and inclusive environments. We can imagine and build communities and a world where we understand each other and foster a culture of collaboration, where everyone's strengths are valued and utilized for the collective good. We all have different strategies and authorities, and this inner authority guides our decision-making. Understanding the spectrum of authority encourages us to appreciate our different decision-making processes, fostering more loving and supportive environments.

From Isolation to Connection

WHEN I FIRST ENTERED THE WORLD of human design and discovered I was a projector, it took me a while to accept having to wait for things. But as I delved deeper into the system of human design, I came to understand that this was my way of being. It would be most beneficial for me to wait to get the best results in order for my purpose to unfold and for me to stay on the path toward my destiny. When some people come into the system of human design, they find they have been going against the grain of how their natural rhythmic energy is supposed to flow in this lifetime. Others have been blessed to be in environments that have already cultivated their aura types in the most organic ways.

Now that is not to say that they still don't have problems accepting and understanding the energetics of their aura type. But what human design does is help with self-acceptance. Human design doesn't mold you into something you're not; it empowers you to embrace your unique and authentic self—flaws and all. It helps you understand why you operate differently from others, fostering self-acceptance and self-compassion. This understanding allows you to make empowered decisions aligned with your natural energetic flow, transcending the limitations of good and bad, and reframing challenges as opportunities.

By delving into human design, I found clarity in my decision-making and a deeper understanding of my relationships. It gave me the empathy to recognize the energetic needs, wants, and desires of others, helping me build stronger, more respectful connections. Despite my personal biases, this framework elevated my emotional intelligence and enriched my interactions with different aura types.

Human design takes us from isolation to connection by offering a framework to understand the diverse energetic landscapes around us, from family to society. Growing up as a projector child among generators, I felt unseen and unheard. Understanding my projector nature made my life easier and more aligned with who I truly am.

Human design is a tool for exploration, not a prescription. It's a multidimensional tapestry that complements your unique experience and challenges the capitalistic approach to success. Each aura type has its own strategy for fulfillment. For example, generators thrive on responding to opportunities, while manifestors initiate action without waiting for permission, making them decisive leaders.

This system shifts our perspective from competition to collaboration, recognizing the unique strengths of each individual. It encourages us to see different types as essential parts of a grand orchestra, fostering synergy and leading to a more fulfilling outcome. Human design helps us move from fear to acceptance, creating a world where everyone belongs. It acknowledges the unhealthy parts of each type, turning shadows into sources of strength when embraced.

Human design leads you to integrate the not-so-good parts of yourself and accept them. You're able to understand who you are in all areas. While you're in the canyon, there is no ignorance or denial of the truth. Human design doesn't allow you to avoid your fears; it inspires you to be more tolerant and accepting of them and integrate them into your day-to-day life. This fosters open space for you to heal and grow.

I must admit that once I started learning more about being a projector, I didn't want to lean in to it at all. I was comfortable living my life as I had been, going after things and, as I say, "trying to make fetch happen." I would get frustrated because I didn't feel like I was being heard by friends or in my romantic relationships. I wasn't finding work I loved. I was stressing myself out so much that I kept hitting brick walls. And it felt like whatever I tried would fail. I was heartbroken by my own efforts. I needed to surrender to the natural flow of my aura. It was hard, but working with my aura type improved my life. I no longer got upset if I wasn't invited to a gathering. I stopped putting pressure on myself when it came to career advancements. I just existed. I learned how to receive and just be in my most authentic flow.

I felt a sense of freedom that I'd never felt before, and it felt good.

Embracing human design at this stage of the canyon leads toward a culmination of your journey of not just self-discovery but also a profound worldview of transformation. It fosters a shift from a world of competition and comparison to one of collaboration and cocreation.

When we embody change, we open ourselves to the pleasures that god / the universe has for us. Human design helped me create change by allowing me to work with my design and not against it. I figured out how to use all my gifts and talents to be who I am and not feel like I am missing out on certain things. I was able to wait for the invitation and be okay with the timing of it all. It also helped me create change in the world by knowing what my greatest strengths are and how to use them to fulfill my purpose and align with my destiny.

The embodiment of change connects you to how you can impact the world and use these embodiments to create your personal legacy through human design. Human design allows you to embody change because it allows you to shift the potential to create a more harmonious, collaborative, and fulfilling world—not only for yourself but for everyone around you.

Integrating the Canyon

IN THE CANYON, HUMAN DESIGN ISN'T just about self-discovery. It's more of a transformative lens that reshapes how you perceive and interact with the world around you. It moves beyond mere categorization to reveal a spectrum of energetic interactions that foster a deeper appreciation for your unique experience and the unique experience that your soul is having as a human. Human design dismantles the idea of fixed personality types. It acknowledges that within each aura type there is a spectrum of vibrant energetic expression that can be influenced by your circumstances, by socioeconomic challenges, and by trauma.

This understanding fosters compassion and acceptance of the different experiences that people within the same aura type might have. You have new tools to appreciate the nuances of people you interact with daily. Understanding your aura type allows you to navigate the world with a greater awareness. It acknowledges the challenges that can arise when you interact with people who are embodying their "not-self" themes.

So how does human design in the canyon create positive change for the world around you—and how does it affect your desire to change the world? It all lies within this embodiment. It's not just about understanding your chart; it's about integrating this self-knowledge into your daily life. For generators, it's not about forcing anything; it's about waiting for your inner yes, for the world to tell you it's time. For manifesting generators, you are here to inform the world after a response and imagine a future bright and joyful. For projectors, waiting for the invitation is not the be-all and end-all; it's about not wasting your energy pushing your guidance and your views and your clarity on those who are not receptive. You are here to recognize genuine invitations and share your wisdom with confidence. For manifestors, this means owning your power and using it with awareness. It means communicating your actions after the fact but being mindful of potential disruptions. It means explaining your "why" to encourage understanding and cooperation from those around you. And for reflectors, you are here to curate environments. Surround yourself with people who inspire and unblock you. Your birthright is taking time for solitude to process any energy that feels off or feels good so you can gain clarity for your own path.

When you are in alignment with your human design, you can collaborate better, spark conversations about social justice, and create movements that others can join. You become a guide for a more conscious world. You offer wisdom to leaders and organizations and people and changemakers around you. You become the changemaker that the world needs. You can dissect decisive action on issues that you're passionate about and inspire others. You can hold space for yourself, for the collective, and for others. You become a mirror that encourages inspiration, introspection, and growth on a community and global scale.

But before you can do that, you have to acknowledge the elephant in the room, which is trauma. That is why it is so important to go through the other embodiments and answer the other questions before you get to this part of the canyon. Your past experiences—especially adverse ones—can shape your energetic blueprint. Past experiences can imprint on us, creating fragmented parts within us that hold on to painful emotions and limiting beliefs. When you understand how trauma might affect each aura type, you can use your aura type to heal and step into your full potential. You have a secret superpower to help you change your world and the world around you.

Your Aura in the Canyon

Generator

In the canyon, you need to imagine yourself brimming with a life force, a powerful engine waiting to be ignited. The essence of your aura is to thrive by responding to life with a deep sacral response. Past experiences of invalidation or pressure to perform can leave you feeling disconnected from your body. You might question your intuition or constantly seek external validation, leading to frustration and a sense of "stuckness." When you ground yourself in practices that can heal you over time, they will reconnect you to your body and your internal wisdom. This is a powerful way to reclaim your energetic authority.

Manifesting Generator

In the canyon, you need to dance to the potent energy that you wish to share with the world. Your intentions in the world are clear communication fueled by your inner knowing of what to do next. You have unhealed trauma that can manifest as impulsive behavior; you may act out without informing others, leading to resentment and misunderstanding. You fear rejection, as it might cause you to hide your powerful energy and to hinder your fullest expression. When you're in the canyon, your goal is to develop assertive communication skills between yourself and the universe. You're here to make your intentions clear. You're here to connect with your inner child and heal your inner child from any rejection, allowing you to express your power in its most authentic form.

Projector

In the canyon, you possess an aura that draws out the best in others. You are waiting not only for an external invitation but also for an internal

invitation. Your wisdom and guidance are so powerful that you need to consider yourself as a lighthouse powerfully beaming and illuminating the path for others, but only when they request it. Remember, your path is not only for others but for yourself as well. You may feel undervalued because of past experiences of neglect or abuse or of not being seen or heard. You may force your guidance on to others, which will lead to pushback and disappointment. At times you may withdraw completely from the world. This causes you to neglect and empower everyone around you. Your goal in the canyon is to set healthy boundaries around your energy. You're here to learn to recognize genuine invitations and differentiate them from people-pleasing tendencies. As you cultivate self-worth and confidence, you will step into your unique gifts.

Manifestor

In the canyon, you operate at a different energetic frequency. Generators and manifesting generators thrive on responding to opportunities and sustaining work. Projectors excel by guiding, and reflectors deeply connect to their environments: You're here to inform others, but you also need to know that informing others may be disruptive. Some people may think that you're domineering or controlling, but you are not—the issue is that some people may act impulsively against you without consideration. You are here to impact others and sometimes that might lead to conflict and isolation, but you are not here to suppress your natural authority. You may feel misunderstood and frustrated, but when you develop emotional intelligence, you navigate the world with compassion. When you know your "why" and can explain it, you foster understanding and collaboration. You learn to read the energy of others to help determine the optimal timing for both their actions and your own.

Reflector

Reflectors are the most sensitive in general, in and out of the canyon. The energy that you absorb and reflect for everything around you is constantly evolving in response to your environment. This can be very overwhelming at times. When you are exposed to toxic environments or emotional volatility, it can leave you feeling drained and lost. You may struggle to discern your own needs and your own desires because you are picking up energy that does not belong to you. You must learn to cultivate a safe container of supportive relationships, nurturing environments, and experiences that surprise you and give you a feeling of joy—this is crucial for your growth. When you learn to disengage from draining energy and prioritize your self-care, you become an essential part of the world around you. When you spend time connecting with your most authentic self, people get to see you for the truth of who you are, inspiring them to be their own truth as well.

Human design is not a rigid instruction manual; it's more like a compass or a mystical map. It is a tool for self-discovery and empowerment.

Think about all the times you forced life to happen for you. Did you feel like you were going against the grain? Did you feel like everything and everyone was against you? Maybe you were just not following your human design strategy, or maybe there was another way to be that you were resisting.

Human design can be very healing in the canyon. When you are in the canyon, your journey begins with recognizing and acknowledging the shadow aspects with illumination provided by your human design. This acknowledgment isn't about judgment or self-criticism but about bringing compassion and awareness to these parts of yourself. Delving into the nuances of your design, you can understand why certain behaviors or patterns persist in your life. This understanding fosters acceptance, which is a crucial step for healing. Recognizing these patterns paved the way for healthier boundaries and self-expression for me. With awareness and acceptance, transformation becomes possible. You learn to harness the energy of your shadow, turning potential vulnerabilities into strengths. As you engage in this profound canyon work, the ripple effects extend far beyond your personal realm, far beyond your relationships, your community, your collective consciousness. By understanding and integrating the work that you do in the canyon, you can approach relationships with greater authenticity and depth. This openness invites others to connect with you more genuinely, fostering relationships built on understanding and mutual growth. Embodying your true self, shadows included, you become a beacon of authenticity and courage, inspiring others to explore their depths. You become a personal leader, and this authenticity transforms you into a more empathetic, inclusive, and encouraging person who can provide effective guidance and embrace others for their full selves. In the grand scheme of our lives, human design offers not just a blueprint of our individuality but also a profound tool for navigating the shadowy waters of our psyche.

Harnessing the Potential of Human Design

OPRAH ONCE SAID, "GOD CAN DREAM a bigger dream for me, for you, than you could ever dream for yourself."

At times, we think we know how things will turn out, but when you embody change, you understand that your highest good is always your first priority. You know that you can only see or receive as far or as deep as you've gone from yourself, but what if there's more? What if your vision is different now that you've healed? This is where human design helps you with your destiny: Human design offers an intricate and nuanced understanding of your innate traits, including those aspects you often shun or overlook in your canyon work. Your canyon work is not just a collection of negative traits or experiences; it is a spectrum of unacknowledged, repressed, or misunderstood elements of your being that, when illuminated, can offer profound insights in pathways to healing.

In human design, your shadows often manifest in your open or completely open centers, where you are most susceptible to external influences or conditioning. In human design, the centers represent areas of energy and consciousness within your body and life. There are nine centers, each corresponding to specific themes such as communication, emotions, identity, and intuition. Defined or closed centers emit consistent energy, shaping your fixed traits while open or completely open centers are more fluid and receptive, taking in energy from others and amplifying it. For example, if you have an open emotional solar plexus, that may indicate a tendency to avoid confrontations or to overly adapt to others' emotions, which could shadow aspects of self-sacrifice or conflict avoidance.

The emotional solar plexus in human design is a powerhouse of energy that governs our emotions and how we process them. It's the center that dictates our emotional waves, our highs and lows, and how we ride them. If you have an open emotional solar plexus, it means you're more of a sponge when it comes to emotions. You absorb and amplify the feelings of those around you. This can lead to a tendency to avoid confrontations or to overly adapt to others' emotions, often to the point of self-sacrifice or dodging conflict altogether. You might find yourself bending over backward to keep the peace, but at what cost to your own emotional well-being?

By recognizing these tendencies, you're taking the first step toward integrating these shadow aspects, transforming them from sources of weakness to wellsprings of wisdom and authenticity.

For a deeper dive into the emotional solar plexus and all the other human design centers, and what they really mean for you, check out the QR code in the back of this book.

As you heal from past traumas and integrate your fragmented self-parts, your human design chart will become a living document reflecting your growth and evolution. Human design is not just about individual transformation; it's about creating a ripple effect that starts within you and exudes outside of you. When you embrace and integrate your shadows, you align more closely with your true nature and destiny. This alignment isn't just about personal fulfillment; it's about contributing your unique vibration to the world's symphony and to the world stage, influencing change in elevation on a collective experience.

Through the lens of human design, you can see that your shadows are not impediments, but rather gateways to a deep understanding of yourself. You will become more deeply authentic by deeply aligning with your purpose, and through this transformation you will invite the world and the people in your world to evolve with you. And it will provide a framework that can influence not only personal fulfillment but also societal advancement.

You are creating ripples of change that extend from the self to the world at large, promoting a vision of a society that you value, a society that you respect, a society that contributes to your individuality and your collective experience.

Human Design for Liberation

Human design is the last phase of embodiment because in order to be open to the possibilities that human design can bring, you have to rectify things within yourself and accept that there is a different way to do something. Many people who come to human design quickly judge that it does not work. They may have learned their aura type in the past but never followed through or inquired further to see how it actually applies to their life, or they felt resistance to the truths revealed. When I meet someone, whether it's a potential client or just a random person, and we get into a discussion about different esoteric modalities, when I bring up human design, sometimes people will automatically say, "Oh, I've tried that before. It doesn't work."

Then I ask them if they had implemented it in their day-to-day life or in their dating life or in their working life. And when they say no, I ask, "How do you know it doesn't work if you haven't tried it?" Just like astrology and numerology and other esoteric modalities that we've discussed in this book, human design is a tool in your toolkit. It offers you another perspective or another possibility for you to embrace who you are and live your most authentic and psychic self. Human design offers a magic that can help you see the world through the lens of your aura types. Human design is perceived as a tool that does more than reveal your energetic signature; it also actively engages with it to solidify your magic. This magic can help you realize and harness your individual potential and strengths. This magic is seen as a way of confirming what you instinctively feel about yourself but might not have had the structure or the language to fully acknowledge and integrate into your life.

Have you ever felt a flicker of magic within you? Maybe it's a yearning to bend your reality or to see the world through a lens that you have never seen before. Maybe you've dibbled and dabbled in different rituals, and you were trying to unlock secrets hidden within, only to find them elusive and not working for you. Human design isn't just another collection of random spells or rituals. Human design is the key that unlocks the door to your own inner magic as you travel through the canyon, making this your last stop. The potent magic is already in your veins.

Human design empowers you to become the protagonist of your own magical story. Imagine a world where every action resonates with a subtle power, where your intuition whispers secrets only you can hear. The system of human design categorizes things into energy profiles, authorities, and intricate gates and channels. This can be confusing, so I won't delve into all the complexities of gates and channels here. Instead, please go to the QR code in the back of this book for more detailed explanations and guides to help you further explore these topics.

All of this serves as an affirmation of your deepest intuitions about who you are. This affirmation helps in cultivating self-trust and can solidify the magic that you bring to the world, the unique qualities and capabilities that can feel like your secret superpowers when you are understood and properly directed.

Deep within each of us lies the forgotten history of our magical lineage. By understanding your human design, you embark on a quest to reclaim your birthright, unearthing the forgotten magic that was passed down from generations. Human design reveals a hidden oracle within you, an ancestral memory. This isn't some cryptic parchment—it's your internal guidance system. It's your voice speaking in the unique dialect of your own inner magic. And when you align with your authority, it ensures that your magic isn't just muttering. It shapes your magic into a potent spell or incantation spoken with the unwavering conviction of a seasoned mage. It becomes the key to unlocking the true power that you hold, ensuring that what is inside of you resonates with the fabric of the reality that you choose to create. Imagine your body just like any magical instrument. Human design reveals a network of vibrant energy channels or secret superpowers to your magic. Human design takes you beyond the present, revealing a deeper prophecy on your life's purpose.

Aligning with your magic, with your purpose, allows you to contribute to a grander design, the design of the communities that you want to be in, so you can cocreate a more magical reality. Human design shifts your place in the world because it gives you guidelines so that, no matter what, you can stick to your own inner authority, your own thoughts, ideas, views, and opinions on what success looks like to you or what peace looks like to you or what satisfaction looks like to you or what surprise looks like to you. Human design offers you a tool and a map to change what you want in your world and the world around you.

Embodying change is trusting, surrendering, allowing, and embracing everything that was and is. Human design is the last step in the phases of embodiment because until you grow through all the previous phases, you will not be able to accept the opportunities that human design can offer you.

Throughout my career, there have been times when I wanted to know when it would be my turn, what I was going to be next. I've spent many years trying new vocations, studying, getting my education, getting certificates, taking trainings and workshops—you name it. But when I found human design—or, as I like to say, when human design found me—and I embraced being a projector, I understood that what is best for me will come to me as the perfect invitation. It is my job to be in alignment with the invitations that I desire. The invitations that I receive as a projector are the ones that will help me stay on the path toward my purpose and allow my destiny to unfold. The reason I'm so passionate about human design is that when I was first starting out in the system, I didn't see anyone who looked like me, so I made it my mission to make human design palatable. I remember watching a man on YouTube who was also a projector talk about how he doesn't look for jobs anymore. Anytime he's out of work, he allows jobs to come to him or for him to be invited.

As a Black woman in America, that made no sense at all to me. All my life I had been told that I needed to be the best, to show up and do my best. I couldn't wait around for anyone to do anything for me. With that man on YouTube telling me to wait around for the right opportunity, I had to shift to understand human design through my own lens. And that's why I tell projectors now, "If you stay ready, you don't have to get ready," in the words of Stoic philosopher Marcus Aurelius. Human design has allowed me to show up and be my most authentic self, so when invitations are presented to me, I can decide what is right for me and what isn't. I can trust myself to know, to be content, and to move on when things don't align.

Human design leads us to be changemakers because it gives us permission to follow our own innate authority by knowing our signature, by embracing our natural way of being. Without human design, we chase things that society pressures us to have, things that our parents want us to have, desires that are not our own and with which we would feel out of place. Human design shows that when you are living in alignment with your design, you become more attuned to your authentic self. You become more attuned to the relationships you want to have and to the career choices you desire. You become more aware of who you are meant to be, and your place in the world naturally will adjust. You will attract different opportunities, relationships, and circumstances that resonate with your authentic way of being.

Aligning with your human design is a form of self-realization that not only affects your personal growth but has potential to impact the collective. When you live authentically and with self-awareness, you inspire others to do the same, contributing to a societal shift that celebrates and accepts the diversity in how people live, express, and embody their unique essence. This will lead to a world where each person's magic is not only acknowledged but seen as an essential part of their human tapestry. It will lead to everyone having a richer and more vibrant experience as a soul in this lifetime.

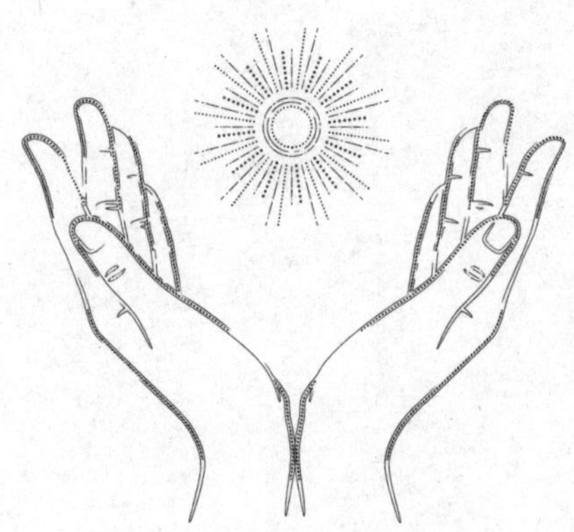

I AM

8

"I AM"

The Embodiment of Destiny

When we talk about destiny, we're basically telling the universe that we're ready to grab hold of what was meant for us. "I AM" is like a deep dive into the heart of who we really are and what we're meant to do. It's about facing the tough, shadowy parts of ourselves—the canyon—and coming out the other side feeling whole and in tune with our real purpose.

I remember my last job in corporate America like it was yesterday. I had just been fired for not meeting my sales numbers. This was not the first time. In one of my earlier sales positions, I remember certain coworkers asking me questions like "What are you doing here?" and I would be confused, not understanding what they meant.

I finally asked a coworker, who said, "You don't belong here. You belong somewhere where people can see your talents and gifts. You're wasting your time here, and I hope you're not here for long."

Deep down inside I knew he was right, but how was I supposed to care for myself? What would I do for money? How would I survive? I didn't have an answer to those questions, and I eventually left that job only to move on to another. I did that for a few years, giving readings on the side, dabbling in various business ventures only to half-ass it because I didn't have the emotional support I needed. I was still building and honing my many crafts with various businesses, everything outside of the one thing that came so natural to me: my psychic and mediumship abilities.

Job after job, I was either laid off or let go. It was as if spirit wanted to put me in a time-out so I could sit with myself and understand that my path was going to be different. I had to listen this one last time. I did, and I never looked back.

My last job became the catalyst for focusing on my gifts in a way that I'd never thought I could. When I was younger, I would see psychics and mediums and coaches use their gifts full-time, and I just never thought it would happen for me because I didn't look a certain way or I wasn't part of a particular group. I was just me: little psychic sensitive Aycee.

Then something happened. I had various incidents where spirit would speak through my body when things were off with romantic relationships, friend groups, jobs, and so on. My body would get an overwhelming rush of emotions, and then, shortly thereafter, things would fall apart—relationships, friendships, or jobs would end. It was the same thing that would happen to me as a kid, the same overwhelming emotional response to the voice of truth inside. And it became my sign to take my gifts seriously and hone them.

I began to build my social media platform and, most significantly, my cherished podcast. My podcast gave me an outlet to speak my truth regardless of whether anyone was listening. I used my gifts and talents to help others navigate through life. I allowed the mic to be the voice I'd suppressed for so long. Today, my podcast is an extension of my heart, a platform where I can express my true self and share my journey with others. It's a space for authentic conversations, deep reflections, and meaningful connection. My gift is helping others play the cards they've been dealt, showing them that they can create their most magical life and be their most authentic self. All it takes is a bit of healing through the trenches of the canyon.

As I journeyed through my own canyon, I found myself at a crossroads of another one. I was doing some deep therapy, unearthing some major things. I was in session with my guides when seven questions and a statement came through me, providing the answers I had been pondering for years.

▫ ▫ ▫

Seven Questions and a Statement

Who am I?

When did I get influenced?

Where can I surrender in my life and allow ease?

What's not aligning in my life, business, or career?

How can I connect to my truth?

Why am I choosing this life?

How do I want to change my world and the world around me?

And finally,

"I AM."

This is not a question. It is both a statement and a declaration of what I am claiming for my life.

These explorations pushed me to go deeper into my healing journey and deeper within my work. These questions led me to write this book.

For years, I ran away from my connection with spirit and with death and didn't want to embrace my mediumship, but I had no other choice. I was called to psychically pick up on the emotional undercurrents of others, especially those who've experienced difficult upbringings or toxic environments or traumatic events. I believe that when we break free from limiting beliefs, we forge new paths toward authenticity.

My own journey of overcoming hardship is now my most powerful tool. I understand pain intimately and can speak to it through my own authenticity. This hasn't been easy at all. It's been a long journey to embrace this.

I worried about what people would say. *Who am I to be a change-maker in the spirituality community?* But the real question is *Who am I not to be?* We all have our destinies. And it is up to us not only to choose them but to become them.

You Are Your Destiny

FOR AS LONG AS I CAN REMEMBER, I existed in a constant state of internal tug-of-war. One side of me craved entrepreneurship, pushing me to start businesses and create and chase wild dreams. The other desperately clung to security, whispering doubts and anxieties about leaving the familiar. The negative voices that ran through my mind stemmed from childhood: being called names by my mother and not being encouraged. These conflicting forces kept me stuck in a frustrating neutral zone. I remained on the runway of life because I didn't have confidence for takeoff.

It wasn't until I passed on an opportunity for an internship that the frustration boiled over. Tears streamed down my face as I realized that fear was once again holding me back. That night, writing the email to cancel the interview, I knew I had to find a way to reconcile these warring parts of myself. I was afraid of being judged—for my looks, my lack of experience, my fears. I had to figure out what was holding me back.

Embarking on a journey of self-discovery, I stumbled upon the concept of Internal Family Systems (IFS) therapy (parts work). The idea of acknowledging diverse internal voices resonated deeply.

Taking long walks in nature, I began a silent dialogue with these opposing forces within myself. I listened to the entrepreneur's yearning for opportunities and the security-seeker's worries about the unknown. Slowly, a sense of empathy bloomed.

I realized that the security-seeker wasn't my enemy; she was a protector shaped by past traumatic experiences. I promised to listen to her concerns, but I also vowed not to let her silence the entrepreneur's dreams. The entrepreneur, in turn, understood the importance of planning and preparation to ease anxieties. With newfound understanding, a shift began. It wasn't a sudden transformation, but a gradual merging. The entrepreneur's spirit started finding joy in exploring new opportunities, while the security-seeker gained confidence in facing calculated risks.

One day, a major opportunity presented itself. With a newfound sense of calm excitement, I realized that the "I AM" staring back at me was different this time. She showed a blend of cautious courage and a thirst for discovery. This "I AM" wasn't about reckless abandon or paralyzing fear. It was about embracing the journey, one well-researched opportunity at a time. It was about honoring all aspects of myself, the dreamer and the planner, to create a life that felt whole and fulfilling.

Saying "I AM" as we grow through this is a big deal. It's like standing up and saying, "This is me, this is my path, and I'm going for it."

It's realizing who we really are, beyond what others say or what we've been through. This isn't just about knowing we're valuable and have something to offer—it's about really stepping into our destiny, living our lives on purpose and for real. It means promising ourselves that we'll stay true to what's deeply right for us, living our lives our way, and showing others what's possible when we embrace who we really are and pursue our destiny. This powerful affirmation of "I AM" guides us toward our destiny.

You can actively call in your destiny, even when it feels out of reach. When you declare, "I AM," followed by positive and empowered attributes or goals, you set a foundation for your identity and your intentions. This affirmation reinforces your self-worth and aligns with your actions and your values and your aspirations, guiding you toward your destiny. The law of attraction suggests that you attract what you focus on by affirming aspects of yourself; in the future, you are more likely to manifest these qualities and experiences in your life steering you toward your desired destiny. Often what holds people back from their destinies are limiting beliefs. When you use "I AM," you challenge and transform these beliefs. For example, changing your self-talk from *I am not good enough* to *I am worthy and capable* can shift your mindset and open pathways to your destiny. When you have a clear sense of your "I AM," your actions and your decisions are more aligned with your authentic self and your unfolding purpose. This alignment helps you make choices that lead you closer to what you want in this lifetime, even when the path seems unclear or challenging.

When you actively call in your destiny, you align with the energy and actions of your goals, and you can achieve great things. At times your destiny may feel out of reach, but declaring your "I AM" helps you maintain faith in your journey. You will always have challenges. You will always have setbacks. They are part of the path. This path teaches you valuable lessons and strengthens your resolve. It allows you to stay adaptable. But by cultivating a strong sense of "I AM," you are not just passively waiting for your destiny to unfold. You are actively shaping it with your beliefs, thoughts, and actions.

When you embrace the journey and trust in your capabilities, you open your life to the opportunities and lessons that come your way, knowing that these are all stepping stones to your destiny. To embody "I AM" is to fully embrace and integrate your sense of identity, your purpose, and your essence at the deepest levels of your being. It's a powerful affirmation that goes beyond mere self-acknowledgment to an acceptance and expression of your true self. The concept of "I AM" is not just about self-recognition; it's an active, dynamic process that influences your thoughts, views, opinions, emotions, decisions, and actions, aligning them with your core values and aspirations. The embodiment of "I AM" is to live with authenticity, intention, and alignment, allowing your true self to guide your choices and actions. This alignment fosters personal fulfillment and growth but also steers you toward an unfolding harmony with your deepest essence.

Embodying "I AM" is not a one-time event; it is the continuous process of growth and evolution. Your "I AM" is your soul's answer to the questions *Who am I?* and *How can I connect to my truth?* As you navigate life's experiences, your understanding of yourself and your purpose deepens your understanding of your soul's journey, rooting it in something greater than yourself. When you continue to refine your "I AM," you incorporate new learnings and experiences. This journey requires ongoing self-reflection, continuous courage, a lifelong commitment to personal growth, and love for this ever-evolving sense of who you are.

Healing All the Parts Heals the Path

IMAGINE YOUR INNER WORLD AS a vast landscape inhabited by various characters—some wise and nurturing, others fearful or impulsive. These characters represent the different parts of you, each with their own unique perspective, motivations, and emotional baggage.

Parts work helps us navigate this inner landscape and build healthy relationships with each of our parts. But what does this have to do with destiny?

The process of healing and integrating our parts is the foundation for discovering and fulfilling our true purpose. When our inner world is fragmented by conflict and unhealed wounds, it's difficult to hear the whispers of our authentic desires and to chart a course toward a fulfilling life. Certain parts, burdened by past experiences, might hold us back from pursuing our destiny.

Through parts work, we can identify these parts, understand their fears, and help them release their burdens. Other parts, like the wise inner guide or the courageous explorer, hold valuable insights and strengths that propel us toward our destiny. This concept is a key component of Internal Family Systems (IFS) therapy, a form of psychotherapy that identifies and works with these various parts within us. For those interested in learning more about the types of parts and how to assess them, I recommend exploring the work of Dr. Richard Schwartz, the founder of IFS.

To begin assessing your own parts, start by reflecting on different aspects of your personality. Notice the inner voices and roles you play in different situations—these could be protector, manager, or exile. Journaling about these roles and how they interact can be a powerful way to gain insight. For a more structured approach, you can read books like *Internal Family Systems Therapy* by Richard Schwartz or seek out resources and workshops offered by certified IFS practitioners.

Parts work helps us connect with our parts and learn from their wisdom. Sometimes, different parts within us have conflicting agendas. As we heal and integrate our parts, a sense of inner peace and clarity emerges. This allows us to connect with our core essence and align our actions with our true purpose. By integrating parts work, we embark on a transformative journey. We not only heal from past wounds but also discover the strengths and desires that reside within each part.

This newfound wholeness empowers us to step into our destiny and create a life filled with purpose and meaning.

In parts work, specifically within the internal family systems model, each part is viewed as having its own perspective, feelings, memories, goals, and motivations. These parts can sometimes carry burdens and extreme beliefs and emotions that they take on because of harmful life experiences. This work brings those parts together into wholeness by healing their burdens and integrating their positive qualities. This allows you to create a harmonious internal system where you can thrive, not just survive.

Embodying Parts Work

PARTS WORK IS THE EMBODIMENT OF all the modalities we explore on our journey through the canyon. Each modality, whether it's astrology, numerology, or mediumship, connects to different parts within us—exile, firefighter, manager, self, and more. By working with these parts through the lens of IFS, we engage with our internal world in a way that fosters true understanding and integration. This holistic approach allows us not only to identify and heal individual parts but also to bring them into alignment, creating a harmonious and cohesive sense of self. It's through this embodiment that we transform our inner landscape, leading to a more authentic and empowered life.

If we were to match each of the questions and the modalities covered in this book to a specific part within the Internal Family Systems framework, here's how they might correspond:

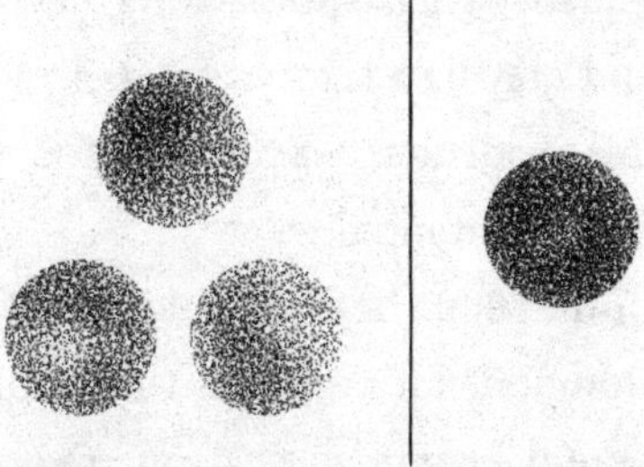

1. **Your Story—Validation (Exiled Parts):** The embodiment of validation is about acknowledging and accepting one's life narrative. The exiled parts are often young, vulnerable parts that carry pain and trauma. They need validation and care to transform and release the burdens they carry. In parts work, this is similar to validating different parts of the self, understanding their stories and the roles they play in your life. Embarking on a journey through the canyon offers a profound opportunity for healing and personal transformation.

   When you begin to validate your narratives, you engage in the acceptance of the exiled parts of the internal family system. These exiled parts are like the hidden chapters of your story and are often laden with the unresolved pain of past traumas or suppressed emotional wounds. There are aspects of ourselves that have been tucked away in the shadows, often out of the need to protect our vulnerability. These parts can carry burdens of shame, fear, or guilt and can significantly influence our behavior and our emotional state in our present lives. When it comes to healing, validation involves gently unearthing these exiled parts from the depths of our shadow. We need to acknowledge their presence and listen to the stories that their pain carries. This is not just about recalling events but about fully recognizing the impact that these experiences have on our lives. For example, an exiled part may surface as a pervasive sense of inadequacy when approaching new opportunities or relationships and may be a legacy of criticism or rejection early in your life. This inadequacy can create a narrative that limits your self-worth and potential.

When we think about healing exiled parts, it is essential to create an environment for ourselves that is full of compassion and nonjudgmental energy so that our pain can be explored and understood. This may involve getting clear about telling your story, asking your family members questions, or connecting with source to get the information you need to validate the stories and honor them so you can transform. The emotional burdens that these stories can carry can be released, allowing them to assume new roles within our lives. And the more we face our stories, the more we can be our truest, most authentic selves.

This process of validation and integration leads to a cohesive sense of self. When you acknowledge and heal your exiled parts, you often find that your self-esteem will improve, your relationships will become more fulfilling, and you will have the ability to navigate life's challenges more easily. Through the healing aspect of your story, you are able to develop ownership over your life's narrative, recognizing that every aspect of your story has contributed to your strength and your resilience. Through this healing journey, the once fragmented pieces of self are woven into a tapestry of a more complete and empowered individual who can move forward with greater clarity and purpose.

2. **Psychic Channeling—Anger (Firefighter Parts):** The embodiment of anger can be associated with the firefighter parts. These parts react to the pain of the exiled parts to impulsively extinguish

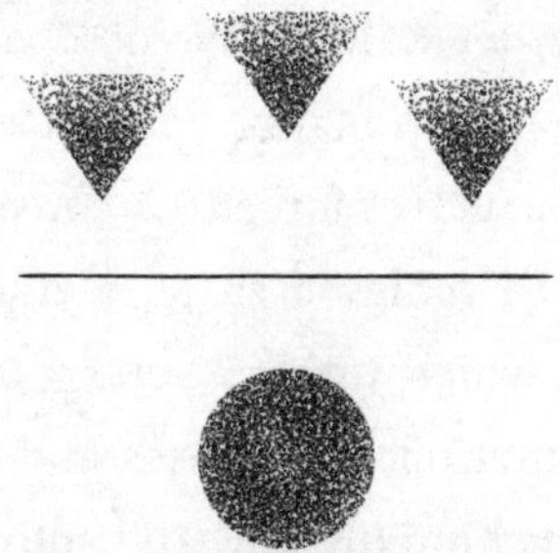

their hurt through behaviors like engaging in verbal arguments, shutting down emotionally, or taking part in risky behaviors. Psychic channeling can be seen as accessing a part that holds anger and learning to channel this energy constructively. Channeling this energy can help you understand the pain that your anger is trying to protect you from.

By engaging with the angry part, you come to understand its protective role and to help it express itself healthily. Navigating through the treacherous terrain of the embodiment of anger in the canyon offers a transformative opportunity as you grapple with the fiery energy of anger. The firefighter parts are categorized by their impulsive strategies to protect you from feeling vulnerable or exposed to underlying pain. They often employ violence or other intense behaviors as a form of psychological armor. These types of reactions can be in response to triggering situations that may serve as a smoke screen for deeper emotional injuries. For example, you might react with disproportionate anger during a conflict not because of the issue at hand but as a defense response rooted in an experience of betrayal or hurt. When I received the UPS box from my ex without warning, it triggered anger inside of me stemming from when I was abandoned as a child in the hospital with third-degree burns.

Healing this part takes you on a deep dive into your psyche to uncover and understand the raw, tender wounds that the firefighter is defending. Psychic channeling in this context refers to the intentional navigation and transformation of anger from a destructive force to a constructive one. Psychic channeling can be achieved through many approaches, such as mindfulness, which teaches you to become more acutely aware of your emotional responses and to pause and reflect rather than to react impulsively, and automatic writing, which can be a powerful tool where you allow your hand to write freely without conscious control, letting messages flow from your higher self or spiritual entities.

When you recognize the early signs of anger, you can start to decode the message it conveys about unmet needs and unresolved issues. Mindfulness and other meditative practices can help you cultivate a space for these insights to emerge. As you learn to channel your anger, you gain access to energy that can be redirected toward self-healing and compassionate communication. You can find creative outlets such as writing, art, or movement that can provide alternative pathways for expressing and processing these intense emotions.

As your healing process unfolds, your firefighter parts can be reassured that they are protected. While at one point they were necessary, after channeling anger the firefighter parts can relax, allowing you to engage with life's challenges with more resilience and calmness. The journey through this part of the canyon can lead you to profound growth. It helps you not only temper your anger but also harness it as a force for personal empowerment and transformation. The goal for you is to reach a place where you can experience and express your emotions without fear or a defensive blaze. This will enable you to cultivate a more harmonious internal environment and healthier relationships with others.

"I AM"

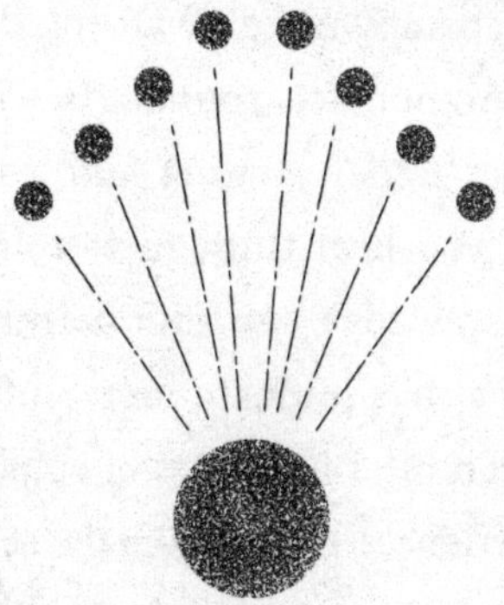

3. **Astrology—Self (The Self):** The embodiment of self can be connected to the self in the internal family system. The self is the compassionate leader and the quality within you that is curious, connected, confident, and calm. Astrology can provide insights into your personality, aiding the self in recognizing and embracing all parts. The spiritual practice of astrology serves as a bridge to the concept of the self, a unique lens through which you can gain profound insights into your inherent nature, your behaviors, and your life patterns. The mapping of astrology can be a guiding force shedding light on your strengths and challenges and the potential paths for your personal evolution.

   In your healing journey through the canyon, astrology empowers the self to step forward as a leader and recognize and embrace the diverse parts that constitute your psyche. When you tap into the wisdom of astrology, it acts as a compass pointing you toward your self's true north. For instance, understanding your sun sign can illuminate some of your core traits, while your moon sign reveals your core emotional needs and how you respond internally to situations. This knowledge helps in demystifying the reasons behind certain reactions or behaviors that might have previously seemed unexplainable.

As the self becomes more aware of these astrological influences, you can approach your parts with greater empathy, fostering a deeper understanding and a more cohesive inner dialogue. When you heal through astrology, it involves integrating cosmic knowledge into your daily life, allowing the self to make decisions that resonate more authentically with your soul. Astrology can offer moments of epiphany where one's life choices and experiences suddenly make sense. The clarity that you gain instills a sense of confidence, allowing you to make decisions from a place of informed self-awareness rather than being swayed by external expectations. This can manifest as choosing a career that aligns with your natural gifts and talents; engaging in relationships that nurture your soul, your value, and your character; or simply adopting lifestyle choices that honor your most authentic self.

Astrology is a powerful tool in the healing process, aiding the self in orchestrating inner harmony among all parts. It can help in healing the fragmentation caused by life's dissonances, guiding you to a place of self-acceptance and self-love. These parts will find their balance under your compassionate leadership, and you will emerge more integrated, resilient, and aligned with your cosmic blueprint.

4. **Numerology—Alignment (Manager Parts):** The embodiment of alignment can be connected to the manager parts in the internal family system. These parts work really hard to keep you functioning and safe. They manage everyday life and work to prevent the pain of exiled parts from surfacing. Numerology offers a path to understand the cosmic design and find alignment in life, which leads to balance and harmony. This is like aligning all parts of the self to work together, recognizing that each has its significant place.

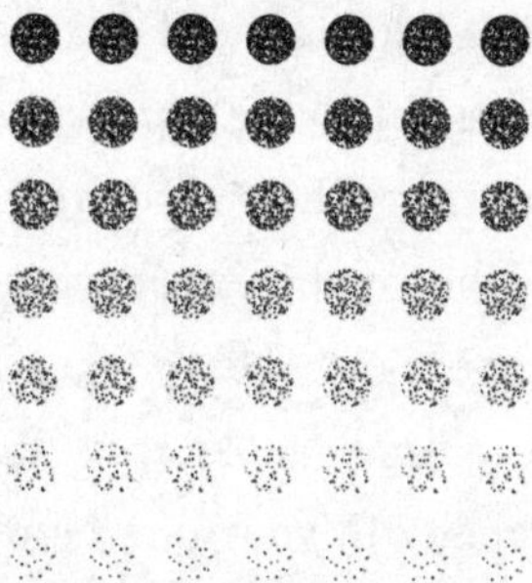

The journey through numerology and the embodiment of alignment is a voyage toward your inner equilibrium. This allows you to engage with the meticulous aspects of your psyche that endeavor to keep your life on a steady course. The manager parts are the diligent inner workers that meticulously plan, organize, and control your daily actions and long-term goals to protect you from harm and emotional exposure. These parts often manifest as relentless overachievers or perfectionists, bearing the brunt of responsibility driven by an underlying fear of chaos or failure.

Numerology provides a complementary method of healing by offering a metaphysical structure for understanding the numerical vibrations that influence your path and your personal characteristics.

Delving into your numbers can reveal tendencies, talents, and life challenges. This offers you a new perspective on why you may adopt certain behaviors. For example, understanding that a life path number can indicate a natural inclination toward leadership and organization might explain your propensity for managerial behavior. When you're aware of this, you start to see these traits not just as strengths but as aspects that need to be balanced and integrated. Healing through numerology involves utilizing these insights to soften the rigid patterns of the manager parts. This can lead to a more authentic and fulfilling life experience, following your natural flow and your core numerological imprint. When you start to see that perfection isn't a prerequisite for worthiness or success, it helps your manager parts loosen their grip. That's when the anxiety begins to ease up, and you can finally make space for a little more vulnerability and spontaneity in your life. Numerological alignment can guide you to adapt more strategies that are less controlling and enabling, giving you the tools to be more graceful and easeful with yourself. Numerology is a guidepost leading to a more harmonious internal structure for yourself. This alignment not only soothes the managerial parts but also liberates the entire system. It allows you to step into your potential with both intention and openness.

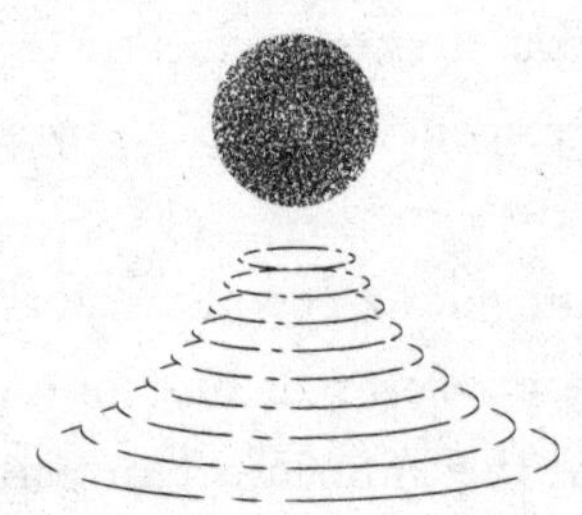

5. **Mediumship—Truth (Legacy Burdens):** The embodiment of truth can be connected to legacy burdens, which are extreme beliefs and emotions that have been carried through family systems or cultural contexts to the present day. Mediumship, which involves communicating with spirits, can be a way of uncovering these truths and beginning the process of unburdening. In parts work, this could be about connecting with the parts that hold different truths or memories, even those that might be hidden or suppressed. The profound passage of mediumship with the em-

bodiment of truth facilitates a deep healing process by addressing the intangible yet heavy loads we carry through our lineage.

Through the canyon, these are the pains, traumas, and patterns passed down from our ancestors, which often subconsciously influence our behaviors and beliefs. Mediumship serves as a powerful conduit to access, confront, and heal these burdens, which are not always apparent in the fabric of our daily consciousness. It offers you a unique form of truth seeking where you as the medium become a bridge to the past, revealing the hidden emotional inheritances that tether you to cycles of suffering. These legacy burdens may manifest as fear, guilt, shame, or self-limiting beliefs that seem to have no direct root in your personal experiences. For example, you might carry a deep-seated fear of scarcity or a pattern of self-sabotage that mirrors the unresolved hardships of previous generations.

Through the practice of mediumship, you can connect with the spirits of your ancestors and uncover the origins of these burdens. You can begin a dialogue that spans across time and dimensions. You can lift the veil to access spiritual communication that allows for the acknowledgment of these traumas and gives you the opportunity to give voice to unspoken stories and unhealed wounds. Healing through mediumship involves not only recognizing these legacy burdens but also actively working to release them. This may involve rituals of forgiveness, symbolic acts of letting go, or just simple acknowledgment of the burden's presence, allowing it to release from your body. Bringing these burdens to light can disrupt the pattern that might be directing your life choices. You can free yourself and those around you to live a life that is not predetermined or preconditioned by the past.

The liberation that you will feel from ancestral traumas

through mediumship can lead to profound transformation, breaking the chains of generational patterns, allowing for a life lived with greater authenticity and greater purpose. The healing of burdens does not deny their existence, but it honors the journey of those who have come before you, enabling you to step into a future unencumbered by their pain. This process can empower you to make choices that resonate with your true self, creating a new legacy of healing and growth and empowering generations that come after you.

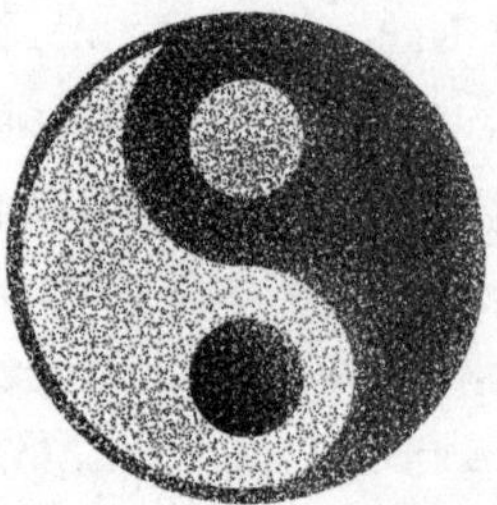

6. **Metaphysics—Choice (Polarized Parts):** The embodiment of choice can be connected to the polarized parts of the internal family system. Polarization occurs when parts conflict with each other. Metaphysics, with its focus on the nature of reality and the power of choice, can help these parts find common ground and reconcile their differences. Metaphysics explores the fundamental nature of reality, including the power of choice, using it to recognize and acknowledge each part to address all needs.

   The journey through metaphysics is an odyssey of reconciling internal conflicts that stem from our diverse and often opposing inner parts. Metaphysics, the philosophical study of being and knowing, provides a broadening perspective through the canyon, illuminating how choice shapes our reality and our personal identity. These parts can pull us in different directions, leading to a stalemate of indecision or a tumultuous inner conflict that stifles our ability to move forward. Healing through metaphysics involves an appreciation of the profound impact that choice has on our lives. This allows us to recognize that even our internal conflicts are a dance of decision-making processes that define our existence. It is about seeing these polarized parts not as adversaries but as aspects of a dynamic system that seeks expression and fulfillment. For instance, you might experience such polarization when considering a career change. A part of you resists because it wants to prioritize financial security, while the adventurous part of you wants to advocate for the pursuit of your passions and your purpose, leading to an internal impasse.

The metaphysical approach to healing encourages dialogue between these polarized parts. This facilitates an understanding that each part has a valid perspective born out of your history and your experiences. Applying metaphysical principles such as the law of attraction or self-concept, you can begin to see how these opposing parts might work together to create a life that honors both security and personal growth.

Self-concept isn't just how you see yourself at your core: your identity, beliefs, and what you think you're worthy of. It's a fundamental principle that shapes your reality. But let's be real: Changing your self-concept, especially through a trauma lens, is hard. In fact, it can feel damn near impossible.

When you've been through some heavy shit, those experiences shape how you see yourself. If you've always felt stuck, broken, or not good enough, it's no wonder that reality mirrors that back to you. The universe doesn't sugarcoat; it gives you exactly what you believe about yourself. And shifting that belief? It's like trying to move mountains with your bare hands.

But here's the thing: Even the smallest shift in how you view yourself can start to change the energy you project. It's not about pretending everything's perfect; it's about daring to believe, just a little, that maybe you deserve better, that maybe you're more than the sum of your traumas. When you start to entertain that thought, you begin to send out a new signal to the universe. And slowly, almost imperceptibly at first, the world around you starts to change in response.

This isn't easy work. It's raw, it's painful, and it's deeply personal. But it's also powerful. Each tiny shift in your self-concept is chiseling away at the old, making room for something new to emerge. It's all about finding synergy between caution and courage; it's all about allowing for life to balance practicality with the pursuit of your dreams.

This process is very introspective, and it can be transformative, enabling you to make choices that are congruent with a deeper understanding of yourself. When these polarized parts learn to negotiate and harmonize with who you are, you accept a gift from the universe. This journey through choice teaches you that conflict can be a catalyst for growth and that it can empower your decisions. And when wielded with awareness and intention, it can lead to a fulfilling, purpose-driven life.

7. **Human Design—Change (Self-Like Parts):** The embodiment of change can be linked to self-like parts. These parts mimic the self and often take on leadership roles, but they do so with clarity and compassion. Human design can help bring these various

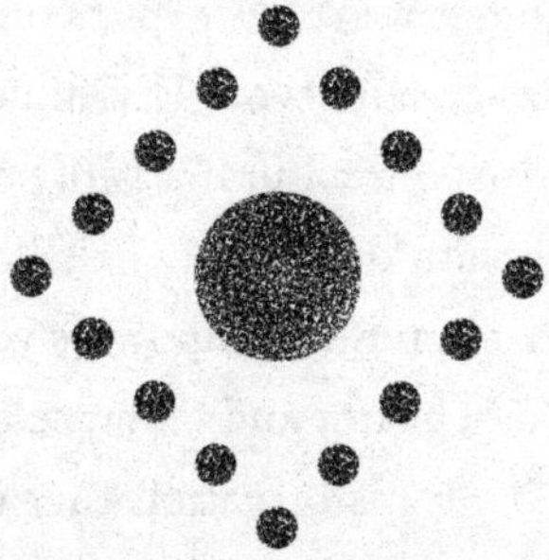

parts together into one's true self and facilitate genuine change and growth. Human design is a system that combines several disciplines to guide personal change. This is about recognizing the need for change and adaptation among the parts to create a healthier system.

The transformative path of human design is like embarking on a profound journey of self-discovery and actualization. These self-like parts, while well-intentioned, may not navigate with the same clarity and compassion as the true self, leading to actions and choices that don't fully align with your authentic nature. These parts might drive you to strive incessantly for achievement or to adopt personas that society deems successful, yet they leave you feeling hollow or fraudulent. This misalignment can lead to a life that on the surface appears successful but lacks a sense of true purpose, true joy, and true happiness.

Human design offers somewhat of a mystical map that helps differentiate the true self from these self-like parts by providing insights into your unique energetic makeup. This system guides you to understand your strengths, vulnerabilities, and potential life themes so you can express yourself authentically. Reviewing your life choices and direction through human design helps you ensure they are in harmony with your true nature as indicated by your human design aura type. This allows you to make decisions that align with your natural way of being and your natural way of interacting with the world.

This process of alignment empowers you to shed those layers of conditioned behavior and embrace qualities of your true self. This leads to a transformation that is not just skin deep but is rooted in the essence of who you are. This is about recognizing and honoring the distinction between who you think you should be, who your family says you should be, and who you truly are.

As self-like parts are acknowledged and understood within the context of human design, they also can be integrated in a way that supports authentic personal growth and change. The result is like a harmonious internal dialogue, a life lived in alignment with your authentic self. This alignment with the true self can release a joyous expression of your unique potential, creating a personal narrative that is deeply aligned with and fulfilling to your true design. This alignment with the true self can unleash a profound and joyous expression of your unique potential.

To embody "I AM" is to stand ten toes down in your existence and in your essence. It is not only a declaration of your presence but also an affirmation of your unique identity. "I AM" grounds you in the very core of your being, holding within it the seed of self-recognition and self-actualization. "I AM" is a powerful acknowledgment that you exist just as you are without the need for external validation or approval.

□ □ □

Your Magical Motherfucking Download

The journey toward a resounding "I AM" begins within. But before we can stand firmly in our essence, we need to address the fragmented parts that make up our inner landscape. This is where parts work comes in.

Imagine yourself staring at a shattered mirror. The reflection you see is distorted, a collection of broken pieces. Parts work helps you gather these fragments—the wounded parts, the critical parts, the protective parts—and begin the process of piecing them together into a coherent whole. Each part, though potentially holding on to pain or limiting beliefs, contributes to the mosaic of who you are. Through parts work, you engage each part with compassion, seeking to understand its motivations and past experiences. Parts that are carrying burdens from the past can dim your inner light. Parts work helps you heal these wounds, allowing them to release their negativity and contribute their strengths to the "I AM" you're building. Some parts, like your exiled or firefighter parts, hold valuable resources. Parts work helps you connect with these parts and tap into their wisdom and encouragement for your journey toward "I AM." Not every part will be sunshine and rainbows. But some of them will!

When we give attention to these hidden parts, we might uncover a deeply buried sense of self-worth and belonging and an unexpected gold mine of creativity and resilience. By acknowledging and nurturing these positive aspects, we can bring them into our daily lives, empowering ourselves to face challenges with more clarity and confidence. The inner work we do leads to a more harmonious and fulfilling life.

As you reflect on these fragments of yourself, certain aspects may stand out. A face etched with worry, whispering doubts, or a defiant scowl shielding you from vulnerability. Take a moment to acknowledge

these fragments. What are they trying to tell you? What fear or unmet need might lie beneath their surface?

Parts work teaches you to navigate even the difficult or challenging parts within, finding ways to integrate them peacefully into your inner system. As you heal and integrate your parts, a beautiful transformation occurs. The fragmented reflection in the mirror starts to come together, revealing a more complete picture of you. This is where the powerful "I AM" begins to take shape. By understanding and accepting all your parts, you gain a deeper sense of self-acceptance. When your inner parts are no longer in conflict, a sense of inner harmony emerges. This allows you to stand confidently in your own power, a core principle of "I AM."

As you integrate your parts, you connect with your essence—your unique talents, values, and desires. This essence fuels the "I AM," allowing you to declare your presence and purpose in the world. The "I AM" is not a destination but an integral companion on your life journey. Parts work provides the tools you need to navigate this journey inward, healing fragmentations and integrating all aspects of yourself. This inner transformation lays the groundwork for a powerful "I AM" that stands firm, grounded, and ready to claim its unique place in the world.

Here's the twist: Imagine another part emerging from the reflection. This is your inner guide, radiating warmth and compassion. What message does this part have for the fragment you identified? Maybe the worried fragment needs reassurance, or the defiant one needs a sense of safety. See if you can find a way for these parts to coexist, even to learn from each other.

Ready to delve deeper? Close your eyes and take a deep breath. Imagine yourself in a calming space within your inner landscape. Perhaps it's a serene meadow or a cozy library. Ask yourself:

- Is there a part of me that feels particularly loud or disruptive?
- Is there a part that seems hidden or ignored?

Focus on one part that comes to mind. Engage in a dialogue with it, just like you did with the fragment in the mirror. Listen to its perspective, its fears, or its desires.

Sometimes, parts hold on to burdens from the past. These burdens can manifest as emotional walls blocking your inner light. Can you identify a wall within your landscape? Now imagine your inner guide approaching the wall with empathy. Perhaps the inner guide can offer the burdened part a soothing balm or a new perspective to help it release its burdens. As these burdens lift, the wall might crumble, revealing a hidden aspect of yourself: creativity, resilience, or a forgotten dream.

Remember, this is your journey. There's no right or wrong way to explore your inner landscape. As you integrate your parts, the fractured image in the mirror begins to shift. The fragments will find their place, forming a more cohesive whole. This is where your "I AM" starts to take root. It's not just a declaration; it's the embodiment of all your parts, strengths, and weaknesses woven together.

Canyon Work Is Shadow Work

YOUR TIME IN THE CANYON IS an invitation to delve into the innermost parts of yourself, experiencing all of your fears and suppressed emotions and unacknowledged desires. As you move through the canyon, you face your shadowy parts, not as an act of confrontation but one of integration, where you learn to embrace all aspects of your being. It is in the acknowledgment of your shadows that you can truly shine a light, not because you have eliminated the dark but because you understand who you are.

The canyon represents your shadow. This canyon is significant. It is not a place to be avoided, nor is it a place that you can bypass until you're ready. It is a place that comes to you when spirit is ready for you to walk through it. By facing your darkness, you unearth hidden strengths and resources. You learn compassion for yourself, and you learn compassion for others. In the canyon you develop the courage to be vulnerable. The canyon is where transformation occurs.

When you enter into the canyon, you do so to clear out all of the things that have been holding you back so you can connect to your soul's purpose and path. Entering into the canyon breeds a fire within you that lets you know that no matter how tough life can get, you have the strength and the courage to move through the canyon with grace. At times, the canyon work will not be easy, but it will not and cannot be avoided. You may have to go through the canyon at various times. It is not a one-and-done experience; it is part of the ongoing journey of life and of healing.

This work through the canyon can be challenging, but know that your soul has equipped you with all of the tools needed to get through it. I feel like I have been through various canyons in my life. My first epic canyon was when I was burned at the age of four. That canyon shaped everything. It was the start of me not understanding why I was different, and it also activated my psychic gifts. When I walked through that first canyon, I spent many years not understanding who I was, and that is because I don't have any recollection of my body before my wounds. Every time I look in the mirror I am reminded of the trauma and tragedy of my burn.

My journey to "I AM" has been one of great pain and great pleasure. At various times in my life, I have realized that the power of "I AM" lies in its potential to unlock a life of authenticity. It lies in the potential to unlock a life of purpose and fulfillment. It is a declaration that empowers me and you to step into our full potential and become active participants in cocreating our destiny. The journey of "I AM" takes you from the shallows of self-doubt to the depths of self-discovery. None of that is linear or easy, and it doesn't come with a manual, even with all the modalities at your fingertips. I've had to accept that I am discovering my most authentic self through trial and error and that I will be on this path throughout my life.

These modalities can help you into and out of the canyon, but you still have to get through. Sometimes, the best we can do is just get through.

Declaring your "I AM" is more than just knowing who you are; it is knowing where you've come from and also being open to where you're going. The privilege of being able to walk through the canyon is an honor that every soul wishes their human body would endure. Some don't even venture into the canyon because it is too scary, but if you are reading this book, you are one of the courageous ones.

The canyon is a spiritual pilgrimage to the heart of your existence, stripping away the nonessentials, the imposed or conditioned identities, and the mask that you may have been wearing. It is about standing out in your truth, claiming your space in the world, and walking in your path of destiny with courage, integrity, and—most important—authenticity.

The canyon holds your unhealed wounds, repressed emotions, and negative self-beliefs, and it requires that you face these shadows. When you acknowledge these aspects without judgment and integrate them into your wholeness, you become more authentic and your light shines brighter. When you claim your "I AM," it is a statement of power. It signifies taking ownership of your life and your choices, recognizing the unique gifts and talents that you possess and have the courage to express in the world.

The canyon becomes a bridge to your destiny. By walking through

it, you do some serious soul-searching and healing, getting rid of old beliefs, healing wounds, and breaking down the walls that stop you from truly shining and following your dreams. Your journey through the canyon is not about a badge of honor but more about your declaration of wholeness and being alive. This life that you have chosen is one that many might not find, but you did.

Your "I AM" becomes a bridge in several ways, clarifying your purpose as you gain self-awareness. As you integrate what you've learned in the canyon, your true purpose begins to emerge. You become more attuned to your inner compass—the voice that guides you toward what you are meant to do. This voice might not always guide you toward something grand or world changing; it may be as simple as bringing joy and happiness to others. For example, think about how a genuine smile or a kind word can light up someone's day. Small acts of kindness not only uplift others but also enrich our own lives. This creates a ripple effect of connection and positivity. The joy that radiates from you will be a by-product of your most authentic self.

But "I AM" also aligns you with your authenticity as your destiny unfolds through your choices. When you embody your "I AM," you act from a place of truth, allowing you to make choices that resonate with your core values and your purpose. This alignment creates flow and a sense of being on the right path. It lets you know that you are ready for the next steps. You can believe in yourself and your ability to navigate obstacles because you are rooted in your most authentic being.

When walking through the canyon, with its winding paths and varied landscapes, "I AM" becomes a great exploration of self-growth, transforming ourselves by dealing with the parts of us that we might not like to look at but that are key to who we really are and can be.

When you proclaim "I AM" from the cadence of your voice, you are not just announcing your presence in the world. You are also inviting the fulfillment of your deepest potential; you are announcing to the universe that you are ready to step into your destiny. On the surface, this "I AM" statement can be deceptive. Yet to truly embody "I AM" is a profound journey that dives into the core of who you are and the path you are meant to walk. It is the unfolding of your purpose and your destiny.

The embodiment of destiny, "I AM" is a call to reach for your best, to handle your inner struggles bravely, and to come out as your true self, ready to give your special gifts to the world. The embodiment of destiny suggests a profound connection between your innermost purpose and the tangible realization of that purpose in the world. There is a deep and meaningful alignment between your purpose and your actual experiences and actions in life.

Destiny is not passive; it is realized through action. Embodiment involves taking consistent, aligned actions that manifest your destiny in the physical world. It's about living your "I AM" in everyday life.

Embodiment is holistic. It requires integrating all parts of yourself, shadows and light, to truly step into your destiny. This means accepting all aspects of your being and using them as strengths on your path. Destiny is not static. The embodiment of destiny is an evolutionary process where "I AM" can grow and expand. As you change and the world changes, so too might your understanding and manifestation of your destiny.

The canyon is not a one-time thing; you may need to return to it at various points in your life. Just know that the canyon can help you become the best and most psychic part of yourself. Your most authentic self equals your most psychic self, and your most psychic self connects you to spirit in order for spirit to guide you toward your truth and your destiny.

I wrote this book because I know what it's like to feel as if no one hears your cries, no one sees your pain—to move through life wounded and healing on your own, time and time again. I wrote this book because I've been through the canyon many times, and on each journey I've learned something new. I've healed another part of me, and I've become a more fulfilled person within myself. The canyon has led me ever closer to the purpose that I am living now, and it will continue to allow me to unfold my destiny.

CONCLUSION

My Embodied Magic and Yours

THE WORLD SHIMMERED.

I'd just devoured the most divine Calabrian chili pappardelle at my favorite Italian restaurant, where my friend and I had been lost in a heartfelt conversation about love. I was gushing about this incredible man I'd met, a connection that felt like coming home. And then came the cherry on top: My agent's text vibrated in my pocket—the book deal was sealed! Tears welled in my eyes, a sweet mix of relief and pure joy. Finally, it felt like my turn.

After years of slogging through the trenches, battling self-doubt, and yearning for a sign from the universe, it had arrived. Those whispers from my spirit guides, the ones that soothed my bitterness when I compared myself to others, echoed in my mind: "Don't worry. Your time is coming, and when it does, it won't miss you." This was undeniably it.

But life, that messy bitch, had other plans. One phone call and a dusty UPS box later, the love story evaporated. The book deal held firm, but my heart ached with the raw sting of heartbreak. Here I was, staring down the barrel of my most challenging project yet: writing a book with a soul laid bare. This wasn't supposed to happen again. I'd entered the canyon of pain before, emerged stronger, and felt healed. But canyon journeys, I've learned, don't operate on a predetermined schedule. They appear when your soul demands a metamorphosis, a shedding of past selves in favor of a more magnificent you. Tears blurred the pages, and my thoughts were a tangled mess of memories and what-ifs.

Yet a deeper truth emerged. The heartbreak wasn't solely about the love I'd lost, but a reflection of the immense healing I'd unknowingly undertaken. It was this very healing that manifested the love and ultimately forced me to choose myself, to remember the scared four-year-old me, lost and alone, suffering from third-degree burns in a hospital room, and offer her the comfort I never received. This was my soul's urgent message: to climb into bed with that little girl, whisper reassurances, and vow unwavering protection.

This heartbreak wasn't about a lost love, but about finally letting go of a version of myself that clung to false security and endless rounds of second chances. The pain was excruciating, but the liberation it brought was unlike anything I'd ever known. This wasn't just heartbreak; it was an initiation, a claiming of my worth. The years spent grappling with self-doubt evaporated. I was valuable, I always had been, and for the first time, I truly believed it. This newfound certainty made me unstoppable. I am unstoppable. And so are you.

This book is more than a gift to the world; it's a profound offering to myself, my lineage, and the relentless evolution of my soul. There are no accidents, only divine orchestration. This heartbreak, this tearing away of an old self, was divinely timed. My body was ready, and though incredibly painful, it was the most freeing experience of my life. And from the ashes, a new me arose—stronger, wiser, and with a heart overflowing with gratitude for the lessons, the resilience, and my unwavering belief in my own worth.

This is my story, a testament to the canyon we don't see coming, the heartbreaks that propel us forward, and the unstoppable spirit that resides within us all. The process of writing this book became a forge, tempering my spirit with vulnerability and self-compassion. I learned to differentiate between healthy introspection and the destructive rumination that had plagued me for years. The book became a beacon, a constant nudge toward self-discovery.

As I delved deeper into the themes of healing and self-love, I unearthed forgotten dreams, passions I'd buried beneath layers of self-neglect. A spark ignited within me, a yearning to reconnect with the artist I'd always been at my core. The love story, the one that had shattered my heart open, became the catalyst for a transformation I never could have orchestrated on my own. It forced me to confront my vulnerabilities, to excavate the parts of myself that craved love and acceptance. In the process, I discovered a wellspring of love within, a deep appreciation for the woman I had become. This is not the ending I envisioned that night at the Italian restaurant, but it's a far more empowering one. I stand here, heart open, a testament to the resilience of the human spirit. The canyon may come, unexpected and unwelcome, but it needn't break us. It can become a crucible, inviting us to forge a strength and wisdom we never knew we possessed.

And from the ashes, a love unlike any other emerges—the fierce, unwavering love for ourselves.

Oracle Is Just Another Word for Teacher

DEEP WITHIN MY CORE LIES the captain of occult—a powerful oracle wielding modalities that pierce the veil and weave together the threads of my ancestral tapestry. Yet this very power I possess often lies dormant, a neglected treasure locked away. It was the canyon, that descent into heartbreak, that jolted me awake, urging me to reclaim my birthright with a clear head and an open heart.

Throughout my life, I'd dabbled in these modalities, each offering a piece of the puzzle. Some seasons required just a single question answered, a nudge in the right direction before I continued down my path of learning and growth. Then the pull to delve deeper would return, beckoning me back into the canyon for another leg of the journey. But this time, the canyon held a different kind of challenge. There was no quick fix, no temporary reprieve. I knew instinctively that I couldn't escape, that I had to confront the work I'd started years ago in therapy—the work of understanding boundaries and truly facing myself. The reflection staring back from the mirror was a stranger. The person I thought I was fractured, leaving an unsettling question echoing in the void: *Who am I, truly? Was the woman I was healing even the woman I desired to become?* The answer, unveiled layer by layer, was a resounding *Not quite*. Yet within the confusion and loss, a glimmer of truth emerged. These modalities, my neglected tools, whispered reassurance. They confirmed not only that I was on the right path but that I was aligned with my destiny. Spirit, it seems, has a way of granting our deepest desires, even when they arrive disguised as heartbreak.

Through knowing my story, psychic channeling, astrology,

numerology, mediumship, metaphysics, and human design, I was forced to confront a harsh question: *What was I truly calling in for my life, in love and in living?* It was an opportunity to claim what served me, what honored my truth and the kindness I exuded to the world. I was living my destiny but was oblivious to that fact. My perspective was mired in loss when I was gaining everything. The unknown, once a source of fear, became the road map. It was the key to unlocking my purpose. Within the canyon's depths, I embraced the unknown as my guide. Knowingness, while comforting, had often crippled me with fear of what lay ahead.

This new approach fostered a profound sense of presence. Each modality served as a safe haven, a space to contemplate the deepest questions and delve into the core of my being.

My channeling deepened, my mediumship intensified, my intuition soared. These gifts blossomed anew as I ventured into the canyon, terrified yet determined. I learned to sit with every emotion that arose, to name it, to feel it without flinching. Healing wasn't about rushing past the pain; it was about diving in and exploring its depths. The privilege of taking this time for myself, nurturing my mind and body while unearthing the most painful memories—both personal and professional—isn't available to everyone. But spirit, in its infinite wisdom, granted me this space.

▫ ▫ ▫

Embody Your Magic with the Help of These Teachers

These modalities became my teachers, reminding me that the choice in how I healed was mine.

- The teacher of validation. I sat with my past, tracing the lines of every scar, every hidden wound. In these moments of reflection, the exiled parts whispered stories I had forgotten. They showed me how each strand of pain could be woven into a tapestry of strength. My story became a cohesive narrative of resilience, guiding me to a place of deep self-acceptance.
- The teacher of anger. Anger surged within me, a firestorm threatening to consume all of my existence. Through psychic channeling, I stepped into the flames and found the firefighter parts guarding something precious: my power. Instead of letting anger destroy, I learned to harness it. I turned that fierce energy into a beacon that illuminated my path forward, pushing me to create change where it was needed most.
- The teacher of self. Astrology revealed that the stars aren't distant. They are mirrors reflecting that vast potential within. Astrology didn't just map my personality; it revealed the constellations within my soul. In surrendering to the cosmic dance, I found where I could ease into the flow of life, guided by the self, who knew the way even when I did not.
- The teacher of alignment. Numerology danced before me, each number a key to a door I hadn't known existed. The manager parts guided my hand as I unlocked each door, revealing spaces within me where alignment had wavered. With each discovery, I adjusted, recalibrated, and found myself stepping back into harmony with the rhythm of the universe.

- The teacher of truth. Mediumship wasn't just about hearing the spirit world. It was about listening to the truths buried deep within me. Legacy burdens, heavy and ancient, rose to the surface. But instead of being weighed down, I released them, each truth setting me free, each burden lifted bringing me closer to my authentic voice.
- The teacher of choice: Metaphysics invited me to trace those threads, to see the polarized parts, conflicted yet intertwined. As I pulled each thread, the fabric of my reality began to shift. No longer was I bound by unconscious decisions. I chose with intention, crafting a life that resonated with my soul's deepest desires.
- The teacher of change: Human design held up a mirror, showing me the self-like parts that had been waiting, dormant, for liberation. With each insight, I began to rebuild brick by brick, creating a life that reflected not just who I was but also the powerful being I was becoming.
- The teacher of destiny. The "I AM" stirred a voice not of words but of pure essence. It wasn't an external calling; it was a force from within, urging me to rise, to embody the fullness of who I was meant to be. With each step, I didn't just walk a path; I created it, fulfilling a destiny that had always been written in the stars but now was etched in the very core of my being.

I finally understood the profound truth: The only way out is through.

The canyon wasn't a detour but a necessary journey on the path to wholeness. It wasn't about skipping steps but about confronting the uncomfortable truths, even if it took longer than expected. When confusion clouded the messages from spirit, the only path forward was to listen, to sit still and receive guidance. Force wouldn't pave the way; only patient receptivity would unlock the next step.

These modalities became my lifelines. They helped me not only navigate the heart-wrenching descent into the canyon but also emerge with a profound understanding of my destiny. I embraced the unknown with open arms, confident in my emotional intelligence and ready to receive whatever awaited me, knowing I am finally equipped to handle it.

I HOPE THAT *EMBODY YOUR MAGIC* has acted as a blueprint for your healing journey, explaining the "why" behind the practices and connecting the dots to help you weave your ancestry into your story. It positions healing as a journey of reconnecting with a larger truth, be it a divine source, god, the universe, or your own inner compass. And it emphasizes that by understanding your personal and ancestral trauma, the layers you unpack can unlock your most authentic and psychic self. This connection to something bigger provides a sense of purpose and direction for the healing process. And this book helps you understand your inner landscape, guiding you on how to integrate those exiled or reactive parts back into your whole self.

Each embodiment is a pathway in the canyon, taking you through emotional healing, navigating life, transforming your reality, and providing a framework for exploration without dictating a rigid path. I invite you to create your own unique path toward self-discovery, a life aligned with your truth, and the activation of your own magic. The book provides the tools and inspiration to build a healing sanctuary, a safe and supportive space where you can continuously grow and evolve on your journey of self-discovery.

Once you've answered the big questions about who you are,

now you get to make a choice about who you want to be. You can really hear what your heart's desires are—those nudges from the universe—and declare who you are going to be in this life.

Each path you choose is yours to explore. You might stumble or have moments of doubt, but remember, you are the architect of your reality. The tools are in your hands, the map etched in your heart. Let your intuition be your compass, your desires the guiding star. This journey isn't a rigid path but a vibrant dance with your authentic self. Embrace the shadows, for they hold the light. Integrate all the parts that make you whole: the exile, the firefighter, the manager. This is where your magic thrives, in the magnificent tapestry woven from your experiences. Remember, this is your story to tell. You are the author, the artist, and the sculptor of your own destiny. Go forth and create a masterpiece.

We are unstoppable. You are unstoppable. And your destiny cannot wait. This isn't the end, my friend. It's the glorious beginning. This isn't just a book; it's a map and a promise of the power that lies within you. May it unveil the layers of your past and, more important, ignite the future you were always meant to claim.

Acknowledgments

THANK YOU, god, for walking with me and hearing me, even in those moments when my voice felt unheard. You listened. Thank you for bestowing upon me the gifts of psychic ability and mediumship. This journey has been rough, but it has been worth every step.

I want to extend my heartfelt gratitude to my mother, father, and biological dad. Each of you played a role in my journey, doing what you believed was best, even when the road was rocky. Your choices, whether easy or hard, shaped the person I am today. For that, I am truly grateful.

To my grandma, my guiding star, thank you for everything you poured into me. Your love is the rhythm that beats in my heart, driving me forward every single day. It's because of you that I learned to trust my visions and embrace the gifts I was born with. Your wisdom still echoes in my life, reminding me to stand tall in who I am.

To my cousins, my childhood crew—thank you for the memories that will always be a part of me. Your constant presence, protection, and laughter made my early years rich and full. I'm forever grateful.

Acknowledgments

To Ms. Tracy, my therapist and truth teller—thank you. You illuminated so many hidden corners of my soul, guiding me to uncover and heal parts of myself I didn't even know needed attention. You taught me the power of doing the work and standing firm in my boundaries, leading me to become the most authentic version of myself.

To Ms. Gina and Gianna at Curio, Craft & Conjure in Charlotte, North Carolina—your space was a sanctuary during some of my darkest moments while writing this book. You held me when I needed it most and celebrated my light as it began to shine. For your support and love and the magic you've created, I am deeply grateful.

To my friends, the ones who've been by my side through the writing process and long before the words even started flowing—thank you. Your love and encouragement have meant everything to me. I appreciate you more than words can express, and I love you from the very depths of my heart.

And to my mentors, coaches, and confidants—thank you for believing in me, even when I couldn't quite believe in myself. Your guidance, teachings, and unwavering support have shown me the way. I am eternally grateful for the light you've brought into my life.

To all of you, my village—know that your love, guidance, and presence have been the foundation on which I've built my life. Thank you, from the bottom of my heart, for being there every step of the way.

And to those of you reading this book—thank you for choosing it to accompany you on your journey. I am forever grateful to share this space with you during your healing journey. It is an honor to walk beside you as you uncover the truths within yourself, and I am deeply humbled to be a part of your path to growth and transformation.

Resources

For all book resources and recommendations, scan this QR code.

Adult Children of Emotionally Immature Parents: How to Heal from Distant, Rejecting, or Self-Involved Parents by Lindsay Gibson (New Harbinger Publications, 2015).

Live Your Dreams by Les Brown (William Morrow, 1994).

The Magical Approach: Seth Speaks About the Art of Creative Living by Jane Roberts (Amber-Allen Publishing, 1995).

No Bad Parts: Healing Trauma and Restoring Wholeness with the Internal Family Systems Model by Richard C. Schwartz (Sounds True, 2021).

Resources

Opening to Channel: How to Connect with Your Guide by Sanaya Roman and Duane Packer (HJ Kramer, 1993).

The Secret by Rhonda Byrne (Atria Books / Beyond Words, 2006).

Seth Speaks by Jane Roberts (Bantam, 1984).

You Are the One You've Been Waiting For: Bringing Courageous Love to Intimacy by Richard C. Schwartz (Sounds True, 2022).

About the Author

AYCEE BROWN is a medium, astrologer, spiritual guide, and teacher dedicated to helping people unlock their most magical lives. Known as the "Voice of Truth" for her ability to connect individuals with their divine source, Aycee works with those at life's crossroads, guiding them to find clarity, meaning, and a path forward. Aycee brings her profound insights in human design and trauma-informed coaching to a wide audience, offering a blueprint for breaking free from conditioning and embracing one's core self.

Aycee's journey began in childhood, when her unique gifts were first recognized by her maternal grandmother, who encouraged her to embrace her prophetic dreams, psychic abilities, and deep intuitive sense. Throughout her life, Aycee has honed these gifts, navigating personal challenges, including growing up in a chaotic household, and using her experiences to reclaim her own magic. As an only child who often felt different, Aycee learned early on how to play the cards life dealt her—skills she now shares with her clients.

Today, Aycee is committed to showing others that they, too, can live in alignment with their true selves and experience the fulfilling relationships they crave. On her wildly popular podcast, *Is My Aura on Straight?*, she offers practical guidance for listeners' spiritual and personal development.

Through her coaching, courses, and speaking engagements, Aycee helps clients find meaning in their pain, move beyond their trauma, and step fully into their power. In everything she does, Aycee's mission is to empower others to see the magic in who they are, embrace their spiritual gifts, and live their most opulently delicious lives.